Second Edition

Single Best Response
Multiple Choice Questions in
Anatomy

Second Edition

Single Best Response
Multiple Choice Questions in
Anatomy

VG Sawant MS (Anatomy)

Ex-Professor and Head
Department of Anatomy
Dr DY Patil Medical College
Nerul, Navi Mumbai

Ex-Professor, Department of Anatomy
Terna Medical College, Nerul, Navi Mumbai, and
Grant Medical College, Mumbai

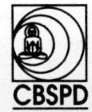

CBSPD

CBS Publishers & Distributors Pvt Ltd

New Delhi • Bengaluru • Chennai • Kochi • Kolkata • Lucknow • Mumbai
Hyderabad • Jharkhand • Nagpur • Patna • Pune • Uttarakhand

Single Best Response
Multiple Choice Questions **in**
ANATOMY
Second Edition

ISBN: 978-93-89396-22-5

Second Edition: 2020
Reprint: 2023
First Edition: 2014

CBS Publishers & Distributors Pvt Ltd
4819/XI Prahlad Street, 24 Ansari Road, Daryaganj, New Delhi 110 002, India.   4819/XI Prahlad Street, 24 Ansari Road, Daryaganj, New Delhi 110 002, India.
Ph: 23289259, 23266861   Website: www.cbspd.com
                                           e-mail: delhi@cbspd.com
Corporate Office: 204 FIE, Industrial Area, Patparganj, Delhi 110 092
Ph: 011-4934 4934   Fax: 011-4934 4935   e-mail: publishing@cbspd.com;
publicity@cbspd.com

Branches

- **Bengaluru:** Seema House 2975, 17th Cross, K.R. Road, Banasankari 2nd Stage, Bengaluru 560 070, Karnataka
  Ph: +91-80-26771678/79   Fax: +91-80-26771680   e-mail: bangalore@cbspd.com
- **Chennai:** 7, Subbaraya Street, Shenoy Nagar, Chennai 600 030, Tamil Nadu, India
  Ph: +91-44-26680620/26681266   Fax: +91-44-42032115   e-mail: chennai@cbspd.com
- **Kochi:** 42/1325, 1326, Power House Road, Opp KSEB, Power House, Ernakulam 682 018, Kochi, Kerala, India
  Ph: +91-484-4059061-65, 67   Fax: +91-484-4059065   e-mail: kochi@cbspd.com
- **Kolkata:** 147, Hind Ceramics Compound, 1st Floor, Nilgunj Road, Belghoria, Kolkata-700056, West Bengal, India
  Ph: +033-25633055, 033-25633056   e-mail: kolkata@cbspd.com
- **Lucknow:** Basement, Khushnuma Complex, 7 Meerabai Marg (Behind Jawahar Bhawan), Lucknow-226001, UP, India
  Ph: +91-522-4000032   e-mail: tiwari.lucknow@cbspd.com
- **Mumbai:** PWD Shed, Gala no 25/26, Ramchandra Bhatt Marg, Next to JJ Hospital Gate no. 2, Opp. Union Bank of India Noorbaug, Mumbai-400009, Maharashtra, India
  Ph: 022-66661880/89   e-mail: mumbai@cbspd.com

Representatives

- **Hyderabad** 0-9885175004
- **Patna** 0-9334159340
- **Jharkhand** 0-9811541605
- **Pune** 0-9923910676
- **Nagpur** 0-9421945513
- **Uttarakhand** 0-9716462459

Printed at: Sanjay Printers, Sahibabad, UP, India

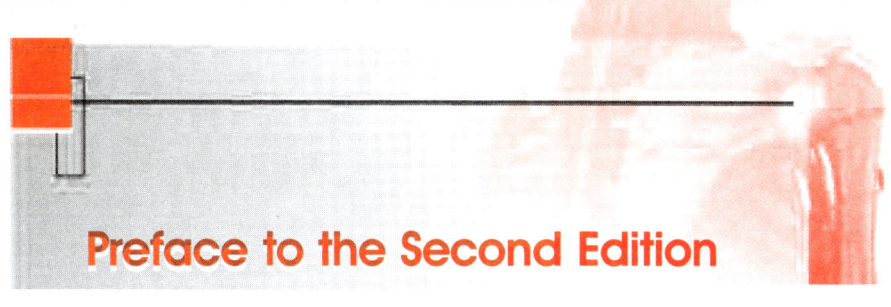

Preface to the Second Edition

It gives me great pleasure to present second edition of *Single Best Response Multiple Choice Questions (MCQs) in Anatomy*. As per new MCI guidelines, topics like medical ethics, embalming, attitude and communication skills have been added in the syllabus. Therefore, new chapters on radiology, medical ethics, embalming, attitude and communication skills have been added.

In this edition more than 700 new MCQs have been added. This book is meant for undergraduate medical students who want to practice after learning. This book is also useful to postgraduate students appearing for various national and international competitive examinations.

I sincerely hope the readers will find this edition interesting and useful. I would love to get fair comments from both the teachers and the students.

I gratefully acknowledge the help and cooperation received from Mr SK Jain, CMD, CBS Publishers & Distributors, and Mr YN Arjuna, Senior Vice-President Publishing Editorial and Publicity. I thank Mr Sarkar, Asstt General Manager, and Mr Javed Hashmi, Area Sales Manager, CBSP&D, Mumbai.

With this I humbly submit this book to the readers.

VG Sawant

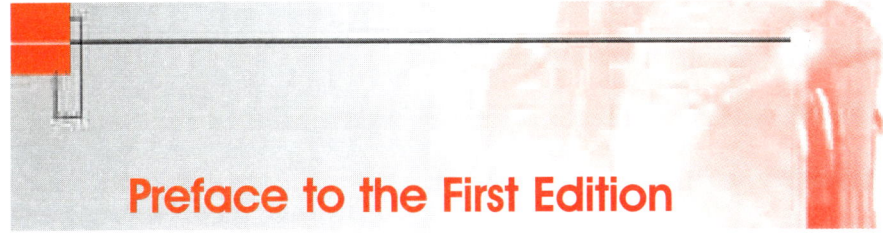

Preface to the First Edition

Change is a part of life. Same applies to the field of education and methods of evaluation. The changes in methods of evaluation from existing subjective methods to gradually more objective type is inevitable. In the process of objective testing subjectivity is totally eliminated. In objective type of evalutation student is expected to choose the correct response out of one or more choices, so his answer is either correct or wrong. This ensures impartial assessment. The objective type of questions can cover wide portion of the syllabus. It also has advantage of ease in correction.

There are various types of objective type of questions, i.e. MCQs, True and False, Fill in the blanks, Matching type, etc. Under new guidelines of Medical Council of India most of the universities have adopted MCQs as tool of evaluation for summative, formative and entrance examinations.

Multiple choice questions are reliable as they are standardized and uniform to all students and eliminate observer's bias. MCQs also test student's ability to recall and to some extent comprehension. MCQs are of following types: (a) Single best reponse, (b) Independent true–false, (c) Multiple completion, (d) Relationship analysis, (e) Matching.

Single best response types of MCQs are easiest to understand and most commonly used in evaluation. Therefore, this book has all single best response type of MCQs. This book is divided into ten chapters. The key is given at the end of each chapter. The students should solve the questions in the forthcoming chapters and get accustomed to solve the MCQs.

My special thanks to Mrs Asha Khandare and Mr Vijay Marathe who had been great help in typing the manuscript.

I thank Mr Javed Hashmi and Mr RN Mandal, General Manager, CBS P&D, for bringing out an excellent copy.

With this I humbly submit this book to the readers.

VG Sawant

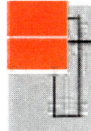

Contents

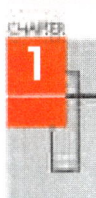
General Anatomy

1. What type of joint is present between tooth and the socket?
    A. Symphysis   B. Syndesmosis
    C. Schindylesis   D. Gomphosis

2. What type of joint is present between ala of the vomer and rostrum of the sphenoid?
    A. Symphysis   B. Syndesmosis
    C. Schindylesis   D. Synchondrosis

3. What type of sutural joint is lambdoid suture?
    A. Serrate   B. Squamous
    C. Denticulate   D. Plane

4. What type of joint is present between basiocciput and basis-phenoid?
    A. Squamous   B. Schindylesis
    C. Primary cartilaginous   D. Secondary cartilaginous

5. What type of joint is atlanto-occipital joint?
    A. Plane   B. Elliposid
    C. Condylar   D. Pivot

6. What type of joint is median atlanto-axial joint?
    A. Elliposid   B. Pivot
    C. Plane   D. Condylar

7. What type of muscle is sartorius?
    A. Fusiform   B. Straplike
    C. Unipennate   D. Spiral fasciculi

8. Fat is absent in superficial fascia of all of the following, EXCEPT:
    A. Eye lid   B. External ear
    C. Cheeks   D. Scrotum

9. All of the following arteries are end arteries, EXCEPT:
    A. Cortical branches of cerebral
    B. Central artery of retina

C. Vasa recta of small intestine
D. Splenic

10. **What type of vessel is an arteriole?**
   A. Exchange
   B. Resistance
   C. Capacitance
   D. Distributing

11. **What type of vessel is vein?**
   A. Exchange
   B. Resistance
   C. Capacitance
   D. Distributing

12. **What type of vessel is elastic artery?**
   A. Conducting
   B. Resistance
   C. Capacitance
   D. Distributing

13. **What type of vessel is muscular artery?**
   A. Exchange
   B. Resistance
   C. Capacitance
   D. Distributing

14. **What type of vessel is sinusoid?**
   A. Exchange
   B. Resistance
   C. Capacitance
   D. Distributing

15. **All of the following bones are membrano-cartilagenous, EXCEPT:**
   A. Occipital
   B. Mandible
   C. Sphenoid
   D. Parietal

16. **What type sutural joint is sagittal suture?**
   A. Serrate
   B. Denticulate
   C. Plane
   D. Squamous

17. **What type of sutural joint is between parietal and squamous part of temporal bone?**
   A. Serrate
   B. Denticulate
   C. Plane
   D. Squamous

18. **Portal circulation is present in all of the following organs, EXCEPT:**
   A. Thyroid
   B. Putuitary
   C. Suprarenal
   D. Kidney

19. **Capillaries are absent in all of the following, EXCEPT:**
   A. Epidermis
   B. Dermis
   C. Hair
   D. Articular cartilage

20. What is the role played by extensors of the wrist in making powerfull fist?
- A. Prime movers
- B. Antagonists
- C. Syngergist
- D. Fixators

21. Which one of the following is an elastic ligament?
- A. Ligamentum patellae
- B. Ligamentum flavum
- C. Anterior longitudinal
- D. Costoclavicular

22. Exagerated thoracic curvature is called:
- A. Kyphosis
- B. Scoliosis
- C. Lordosis
- D. Kyphoscoliosis

23. Exagerated lumbar curvature is called:
- A. Kyphosis
- B. Scoliosis
- C. Lordosis
- D. Kyphoscoliosis

24. In relation to which one of the following vertebra centre of gravity lies in standing position?
- A. Body of 1st lumbar
- B. 2 cm behind the 3rd lumbar
- C. Body of 1st sacral
- D. 2 cm in front the 1st sacral

25. What type of bursa is subscapularis bursa?
- A. Communicating
- B. Non-communicating
- C. Sub-fascial
- D. Subcutaneous

26. All of the following muscles have twisted fasciculi, EXCEPT:
- A. Pectoralis major
- B. Teres minor
- C. Supinator
- D. Trapezius

27. What type of epiphysis is head of the femur?
- A. Pressure
- B. Traction
- C. Atavistic
- D. Aberrant

28. What type of epiphysis is coracoid process of the scapula?
- A. Pressure
- B. Traction
- C. Atavistic
- D. Aberrant

29. What type of epiphysis is lesser trochanter of the femur?
- A. Pressure
- B. Traction
- C. Atavistic
- D. Aberrant

30. What type of epiphysis is greater tubercle of the humerus?
- A. Pressure
- B. Traction
- C. Atavistic
- D. Aberrant

31. What type of epiphysis is lower end of the femur?
- A. Pressure
- B. Traction
- C. Atavistic
- D. Aberrant

32. What type of epiphysis is upper end of the tibia?
- A. Pressure
- B. Traction
- C. Atavistic
- D. Aberrant

33. Which one of the following joints is an ellipsoid joint?
- A. Wrist
- B. Knee
- C. Ankle
- D. Shoulder

34. All of the following muscles have pulley, EXCEPT:
- A. Digastric
- B. Omohyoid
- C. Superior oblique of eye
- D. Stylohyoid

35. What type of synovial joint is the 1st carpometacarpal joint?
- A. Hinge
- B. Saddle
- C. Ellipsoid
- D. Plane

36. What type of joint is the manubriosternal joint?
- A. Saddle
- B. Plane synovial
- C. Symphysis
- D. Syndesmosis

37. Which one of the following joints is saddle joint?
- A. Carpometacarpal joint of thumb
- B. Elbow
- C. Ankle
- D. Knee

38. Which one of the following joints is syndesmosis type of joint?
- A. Sacroiliac
- B. Inferior tibiofibular
- C. Superior tibiofibular
- D. Mid tarsal

39. Which type of epiphysisis Ostrigonum?
- A. Pressure
- B. Traction
- C. Atavistic
- D. Aberrant

40. What type of bone is maxilla?
- A. Short
- B. Sesamoid
- C. Pneumatic
- D. Flat

41. What type of bone is patella?
- A. Short
- B. Sesamoid
- C. Pneumatic
- D. Flat

42. What type of bone is parietal?
    A. Irregular   B. Flat
    C. Pneumatic   D. Short

43. What type of bone is rib?
    A. Irregular   B. Flat
    C. Modified long   D. Short

44. Which muscle is straplike with tendinous intersections?
    A. Rectus femoris   B. Rectus abdominis
    C. Medial rectus   D. Superior rectus

45. What type of bone is occipital bone?
    A. Cartilagenous   B. Membranous
    C. Membrano-cartilagenous D. None of the above

46. What type of muscle is deltoid?
    A. Unipennate   B. Bipennate
    C. Multipennate   D. Circumpennate

47. What type of muscle is flexor pollicis longus?
    A. Unipennate   B. Bipennate
    C. Multipennate   D. Circumpennate

48. What type of muscle is tibialis anterior?
    A. Unipennate   B. Bipennate
    C. Multipennate   D. Circumpennate

49. What type of muscle is biceps brachii?
    A. Straplike   B. Fusiform
    C. Quadrilateral   D. Cruciate

50. What type of muscle is thyrohyoid?
    A. Straplike   B. Fusiform
    C. Quadrilateral   D. Cruciate

51. Which muscle has twisted fasciculi?
    A. Pectoralis major   B. Latissimus dorsi
    C. Trapezius   D. All of the above

52. What type of sutural joint is present between palatine processes of maxilla?
    A. Schindylesis   B. Serrate
    C. Denticulate   D. Plane

53. Which muscle is an example of cruciate muscle?
- A. Sternocleidomastoid
- B. Masseter
- C. Adductor magnus
- D. All of the above

54. What type of neurons are present in dorsal root ganglia?
- A. Unipolar
- B. Bipolar
- C. Pseudounipolar
- D. Multipolar

55. What type of neurons is present in olfactory mucosa?
- A. Unipolar
- B. Bipolar
- C. Pseudounipolar
- D. Multipolar

56. What type of bursa is prepatellar bursa?
- A. Communicating
- B. Submuscular
- C. Subfascial
- D. Subcutaneous

57. What type of bursa is suprapatellar bursa?
- A. Communicating
- B. Non-communicating
- C. Subfascial
- D. Subcutaneous

58. All of the following are traction epiphyses, EXCEPT:
- A. Mastoid process
- B. Greater tronchanter of femur
- C. Epicondyles of humerus
- D. Condyles of tibia

59. What type of bone is a metacarpal?
- A. Long
- B. Short
- C. Modified long
- D. Long short

60. What type of bone is a scaphoid?
- A. Flat
- B. Short
- C. Long short
- D. Sesamoid

61. What type of joint is sternoclavicular joint?
- A. Complex
- B. Saddle
- C. Compound
- D. All of the above

62. What type of joint is pubic symphysis?
- A. Plane synovial
- B. Syndesmosis
- C. Primary cartilaginous
- D. Secondary cartilagenous

63. What is the role of brachialis during flexion of the elbow joint?
- A. Prime mover
- B. Antagonist
- C. Fixator
- D. Synergist

64. What is the role of triceps brachii during flexion of the elbow joint?
    A. Prime mover
    B. Antagonist
    C. Fixator
    D. Synergist

65. Exagerated lateral thoracic curvature is called:
    A. Kyphosis
    B. Scoliosis
    C. Lordosis
    D. Kyphoscoliosis

66. All of the following are modifications of the deep fascia, EXCEPT:
    A. Epicranial aponeurosis
    B. Palmar aponeurosis
    C. Epimysium
    D. External oblique aponeurosis

67. All of the following are pecularities of a sesamoid bone, EXCEPT:
    A. Develops in tendon
    B. Ossifies after birth
    C. Presence of periosteum
    D. Absence of Haversian system

68. All of the following ligaments are largely composed of elastic fibers, EXCEPT:
    A. Ligamentum nuchae
    B. Ligamentum flavum
    C. Spring
    D. Anterior longitudinal

69. Which is the smallest bone in the body?
    A. Pisiform
    B. Malleus
    C. Incus
    D. Stapes

70. Which is the smallest joint in the body?
    A. Incudostapedial
    B. Incudomalleolar
    C. Cricoaryteniod
    D. Cricothyroid

71. All of the following are present in the superficial fascia, EXCEPT:
    A. Platysma
    B. Mammary glands
    C. Bodies of sweat glands
    D. Sebaceous glands

72. In which one of the following, superficial fascia shows stratification (two layers)?
    A. Face
    B. Neck
    C. Upper limb
    D. Anterior abdominal wall

73. What type of joint is the elbow joint?
    A. Plane
    B. Uniaxial
    C. Biaxial
    D. Multiaxial

74. **What type of joint is the superior radio-ulnar joint?**
    A. Plane
    B. Uniaxial
    C. Biaxial
    D. Multiaxial

75. **Around which axis movements of adduction and abduction take place?**
    A. Vertical
    B. Transverse
    C. Antero-posterior
    D. Oblique

76. **Around which axis movements are produced at the elbow joint?**
    A. Vertical
    B. Transverse
    C. Antero-posterior
    D. Oblique

77. **Pump handle movements of the ribs are produced around which axis?**
    A. Vertical
    B. Transverse
    C. Antero-posterior
    D. Oblique

78. **Bucket handle movements of the ribs are produced around which axis?**
    A. Vertical
    B. Transverse
    C. Antero-posterior
    D. Oblique

79. **Which is the largest joint in the body?**
    A. Shoulder
    B. Hip
    C. Knee
    D. Sacroiliac

80. **Around which axis movements are permitted in the pivot joint?**
    A. Vertical
    B. Transverse
    C. Antero-posterior
    D. Oblique

81. **All of the following are tortuous arteries, EXCEPT:**
    A. Nutrient
    B. Uterine
    C. Splenic
    D. Superior mesenteric

82. **What type of joint is the wrist joint?**
    A. Plane
    B. Uniaxial
    C. Biaxial
    D. Multiaxial

83. **What type of joint is the knee joint?**
    A. Plane
    B. Uniaxial
    C. Biaxial
    D. Multiaxial

84. What type of joint is the calcaneocuboid joint?
    A. Plane   B. Uniaxial
    C. Biaxial   D. Multiaxial

85. What type of joint is the first carpometacarpal joint?
    A. Plane   B. Uniaxial
    C. Biaxial   D. Multiaxial

86. What type of joint is the intercarpal joint?
    A. Plane   B. Uniaxial
    C. Biaxial   D. Multiaxial

87. Which arteries form hairpin bends before fusion of epiphyseal plates?
    A. Periosteal   B. Nutrient
    C. Metaphyseal   D. Epiphyseal

88. Around which axis movements of flexion and extension take place?
    A. Vertical   B. Transverse
    C. Antero-posterior   D. Oblique

89. Around which axis movements of medial and lateral rotation take place?
    A. Vertical   B. Transverse
    C. Antero-posterior   D. Oblique

90. What type of joint is present between superior and inferior articular processes of vertebrae?
    A. Plane   B. Uniaxial
    C. Biaxial   D. Multiaxial

91. All of the following are complex joints, EXCEPT:
    A. Temporomandibular   B. Sternoclavicular
    C. Acromioclavicular   D. Knee

92. All of the following are compound joints, EXCEPT:
    A. Elbow   B. Wrist
    C. First carpometacarpal   D. Ankle

93. In articulating surfaces all of the following joints are covered by fibrocartilages, EXCEPT:
    A. Shoulder   B. Sternoclavicular
    C. Acromioclavicular   D. Temporomandibular

94. Which one of the following structural components of a bone, is responsible for its tensile strength?
    A. Hydroxyapatite
    B. Osteonectin
    C. Osteocytes
    D. Collagen fibers

95. In which part of a developing bone, primary center of ossification appears?
    A. Epiphysis
    B. Diaphysis
    C. Metaphysis
    D. Epiphyseal plate

96. In which part of a developing bone, secondary center of ossification appears?
    A. Epiphysis
    B. Diaphysis
    C. Metaphysis
    D. Epiphyseal plate

97. All of the following are fibrous joints, EXCEPT:
    A. Schindylesis
    B. Syndesmoses
    C. Symphysis
    D. Gomphosis

98. Fracture passing through which one of the following may disrupt linear growth of a long bone?
    A. Epiphysis
    B. Epiphyseal plate
    C. Diaphysis
    D. Metaphysis

99. Which one of the following bones has thickest articular carticular in the body?
    A. Lower end of femur
    B. Upper end of tibia
    C. Head of humerus
    D. Patella

100. Sweat glnands are absent over the skin of the following, EXCEPT:
    A. Palm
    B. Margins of lips
    C. Glans penis
    D. Tympanic membrane

101. All of the following muscles represent the panniculus carnosus, EXCEPT:
    A. Platysma
    B. Corrugator cutis
    C. Palmaris brevis
    D. Plantaris

102. All of the following structures are lined by synovial membrane, EXCEPT:
    A. Articular cartilage
    B. Intracapsular tendons
    C. Inner aspect of joint capsule
    D. Intracapsular non-articulating parts of bones

103. What type joint is present between epiphysis and diaphysis?
- A. Fibrous
- B. Primary cartilaginous
- C. Secondary cartilaginous
- D. Synovial

104. All of the following structures contain both skeletal and smooth muscles, EXCEPT:
- A. Middle third of oesophagus
- B. Anal sphincter
- C. Upper eyelid
- D. Tongue

105. Which one of the following structures has maximum blood supply?
- A. Cartilages
- B. Bones
- C. Ligaments
- D. Tendons

106. Which one of the following is supplied by vasa vasorum?
- A. Tunica media and tunica intima
- B. Tunica adventitia and tunica media
- C. Tunica adventita
- D. Tunica adventitia and outer part of tunica media

107. Which one of the following has both afferent and efferent lymphatics?
- A. Spleen
- B. Thymus
- C. Tonsil
- D. Lymph node

108. Which one of the following forms nerve plexuses?
- A. Ventral roots
- B. Dorsal roots
- C. Ventral rami
- D. Dorsal rami

109. All of the following are components of a myelinated nerve fiber, EXCEPT:
- A. Axon
- B. Myelin sheath
- C. Neurilemmal sheath
- D. Epineurium

110. Which one of the following forms neurilemmal sheath?
- A. Schwann's cell cytoplasm
- B. Schwann's cell plasma membrane
- C. Lipids
- D. Endoneurium

111. **From the lateral horns of which of the following spinal segments thoracolumbar outflow arises?**
     A. T1–L1
     B. T1–L2
     C. T1–L3
     D. T1–L5

112. **All of the following are appendages of the skin, EXCEPT:**
     A. Nails
     B. Hair
     C. Sebaceous glands
     D. Arrector pilorum muscles

Superior Extremity

1. What type of joint is sternoclavicular joint?
- A. Plane
- B. Saddle
- C. Ellipsoid
- D. Ball and socket

2. What type of joint is acromioclavicular joint?
- A. Plane
- B. Saddle
- C. Ellipsoid
- D. Ball and socket

3. Brachial plexus is usually formed by ventral rami of which spinal nerves?
- A. C3, C4, C5, C6, C7
- B. C4, C5, C6, C7, C8
- C. C5, C6, C7, C8, T1
- D. C6, C7, C8, T1, T2

4. What type of epiphysis is coracoid process of scapula?
- A. Pressure
- B. Traction
- C. Atavistic
- D. Aberrant

5. What type of bone is clavicle?
- A. Typical long
- B. Modified long
- C. Flat
- D. Miniature long

6. What type of muscle is deltoid?
- A. Unipennate
- B. Bipennate
- C. Multipennate
- D. Circumpennate

7. What is the role of triceps brachii during elbow flexion?
- A. Prime mover
- B. Antagonist
- C. Fixator
- D. Synergist

8. Lymphatics of the medial side of hand and forearm drain into which group of axillary lymph nodes?
- A. Lateral
- B. Posterior
- C. Anterior
- D. Central

9. Adduction of the shoulder joint is carried out by which muscle?
- A. Latssimus dorsi
- B. Deltoid anteior and posterior fibres

C. Pectoralis major

D. All of the above

10. **Which muscle is supplied by suprascapular nerve?**
    A. Rhomboideus major   B. Infraspinatus
    C. Pectoralis major   D. All of the above

11. **What type of joint is wrist joint?**
    A. Condylar   B. Plane
    C. Ellipsoid   D. Saddle

12. **Wrist drop deformity occurs due to damage of which nerve?**
    A Radial   B. Median
    C Ulnar   D. Musculocutaneous

13. **Which artery gives branch accompanying the median nerve?**
    A. Ulnar   B. Radial
    C. Brachial   D. Anterior interosseous

14. **All of the following muscles are attached to greater tuberosity of the humerus, EXCEPT:**
    A. Supraspinatus   B. Infraspinatus
    C. Teres minor   D. Subscapularis

15. **Which muscle is supplied by median nerve in the arm?**
    A. Brachialis   B. Coracobrachialis
    C. Teres minor   D. None of the above

16. **Winging of scapula results from injury to which nerve?**
    A. Suprascapular   B. Subscapular
    C. Long thoracic   D. Axillary

17. **Which structure passes through the carpal tunnel?**
    A. Ulnar artery   B. Ulnar nerve
    C. Radial artery   D. Median nerve

18. **In which one of the following positions dislocation of head of the humerus at the shoulder joint is most common?**
    A. Anteriorly   B. Posteriorly
    C. Superiorly   D. Inferiorly

19. **Which muscle is attached to lesser tuberosity of the humerus?**
    A. Subscapularis   B. Supraspinatus
    C. Teres major   D. Teres minor

20. Axillary nerve passes through which space?
    A. Suprascapular
    B. Upper triangular
    C. Lower triangular
    D. Quadrangular

21. Which spinal nerve supplies the skin of the little finger?
    A. C6
    B. C7
    C. C8
    D. T1

22. All of the following are contents of the cubital fossa, EXCEPT:
    A. Median nerve
    B. Radial nerve
    C. Ulnar nerve
    D. Bicipital aponeurosis

23. What type of muscle is flexor pollicis longus?
    A. Unipennate
    B. Bipennate
    C. Multipennate
    D. Circumpennate

24. What type of joint is middle radio-ulnar joint?
    A. Pivot
    B. Hinge
    C. Syndesmosis
    D. None of the above

25. All are the following nerves are branches of the posterior cord of brachial plexus, EXCEPT:
    A. Ulnar
    B. Radial
    C. Axillary
    D. Upper subscapular

26. Which muscle is supplied by axillary nerve?
    A. Pectoralis minor
    B. Pectoralis major
    C. Teres minor
    D. Teres major

27. From which part of brachial plexus does the long thoracic nerve (nerve to serratus anterior) arises?
    A. Roots
    B. Trunks
    C. Divisions
    D. Cords

28. Painful arc syndrome is characterized by pain in which range (in degree) of abduction of the shoulder joint?
    A. 30 to 60
    B. 60 to 120
    C. 90 to 120
    D. 120 to 150

29. Teres major is supplied by which nerve?
    A. Axillary
    B. Radial
    C. Musculocutaneous
    D. Lower subscapular

30. What type of joint is superior radio-ulnar joint?
    A. Condylar
    B. Pivot
    C. Fibrous
    D. Ellipsoid

31. **Which nerve supplies pectoralis major muscle?**
    A. Medial pectoral
    B. Lateral pectoral
    C. Both medial and lateral pectoral
    D. Long thoracic

32. **In carpal tunnel syndrome, which nerve is most likely to be involved?**
    A. Ulnar
    B. Radial
    C. Median
    D. Anterior interosseous

33. **In which one of the following brachioradialis is inserted?**
    A. Base of 1st metacarpal
    B. Base of 2nd metacarpal
    C. Styloid process of ulna
    D. Styloid process of radius

34. **In fracture of medial epicondyle of humerus, which nerve is most likely to be injured?**
    A. Ulnar
    B. Median
    C. Radial
    D. Medical cutaneous nerve of forearm

35. **All of the following muscles have dual nerve supply, EXCEPT:**
    A. Pectoralis major
    B. Brachialis
    C. Pronator teres
    D. Flexor digitorum profundus

36. **What type of joint is carpometacarpal joint of the thumb?**
    A. Condylar
    B. Saddle
    C. Hinge
    D. Plane

37. **At the level of which thoracic vertebra the root of the spine of scapula lies?**
    A. 2
    B. 3
    C. 4
    D. 5

38. **Which one of the following is an example of multipennate muscle?**
    A. Subscapularis
    B. Pornator teres
    C. Subclavius
    D. Triceps

39. **What is the root value of the axillary nerve?**
    A. C5, C6
    B. C5, C6, C7
    C. C5, C6, C7, C8
    D. C5, C6, C7, C8, T1

40. **What is the root value of the long thoracic nerve?**
    A. C3, C4, C5
    B. C4, C5, C6
    C. C5, C6, C7
    D. C6, C7, C8

41. Clavipectoral fascia is pierced by which vein?
   A. Cephalic   B. Axillary
   C. Basilic   D. Median cubital

42. Nerve to subclavius arises from which part of brachial plexus?
   A. Roots   B. Trunk
   C. Division   D. Cord

43. Brachioradialis is an example of which type of muscle?
   A. Swing   B. Spin.
   C. Spindle   D. Shunt

44. Lateral two lumbricals are supplied by which nerve?
   A. Ulnar   B. Median
   C. Radial   D. Axillary

45. Lateral cutaneous nerve of foramen is a branch of which nerve?
   A. Ulnar   B. Median
   C. Radial   D. Musculocutaneous

46. All of the following nerves are in contact with the humerus, EXCEPT:
   A. Ulnar   B. Median
   C. Radial   D. Axillary

47. Which nerve supplies medial half of flexor digitorum profundus muscle?
   A. Ulnar   B. Median
   C. Radial   D. Musculocutaneous

48. Which nerve lies in the quadrangular space of the arm?
   A. Ulnar   B. Median
   C. Radial   D. Axillary

49. Which nerve supplies brachialis muscle?
   A. Ulnar
   B. Musculocutaneous
   C. Median
   D. Axillary

50. Inability to oppose the thumb to the little finger can result from damage to which nerve?
   A. Ulnar   B. Radial
   C. Median   D. Axillary

51. What is the root value of musculocutaneous nerve?
  A. C4, C5
  B. C5, C6, C7
  C. C5, C6, C7, C8
  D. C8, T1

52. To which structure the medial collateral ligament of the elbow joint is closely related?
  A. Ulnar nerve
  B. Brachial artery
  C. Radial nerve
  D. Ulnar artery

53. Which is the first bone to ossify in the body?
  A. Clavicle
  B. Scapula
  C. Mandible
  D. Humerus

54. How many lactiferous ducts are present in each breast?
  A. 1
  B. 10
  C. 10–15
  D. 15–20

55. Due to partial tearing or degeneration of which one of the following causes Golfer's elbow?
  A. Common flexor origin
  B. Common extensor origin
  C. Pronator teres
  D. Supinator

56. Due to partial tearing or degeneration of which one of the following causes tennis elbow?
  A. Common flexor origin
  B. Common extensor origin
  C. Cubital fossa
  D. Olecranon process

57. From which part of brachial plexus does the suprascapular nerve arises?
  A. Roots
  B. Trunks
  C. Divisions
  D. Cords

58. Which is the site of injury to brachial plexus in Erb's paralysis?
  A. Lateral cord
  B. Lower trunk
  C. Upper trunk
  D. Middle trunk

59. Which muscle is supplied by the ulnar nerve?
  A. Supinator
  B. 1st lumbrical
  C. Opponens pollicis
  D. Adductor pollicis

60. Which muscle is supplied by lower subscapular nerve?
  A. Teres minor
  B. Teres major
  C. Subclavius
  D. Supraspinatus

61. **Medial cord of the brachial plexus lies medial to which structure?**
    A. Axillary vein   B. Axillary artery
    C. Serratus anterior   D. Pectoralis major

62. **The mammary gland drains into following axillary group of lymph nodes, EXCEPT:**
    A. Anterior   B. Lateral
    C. Central   D. Apical

63. **Paralysis of upper trunk of brachial plexus results in which deformity?**
    A. Ape hand   B. Clawhand
    C. "Waiter tip" hand   D. Winged scapula

64. **All of the following muscles are supplied by the musculo-cutaneous nerve, EXCEPT:**
    A. Coracobrachialis   B. Biceps brachii
    C. Brachialis   D. Brachioradialis

65. **What type of muscle is biceps brachii?**
    A. Unipennate   B. Bipennate
    C. Multipennate   D. Fusiform

66. **In which vein does the cephalic vein drain?**
    A. Subclavian   B. Axillary
    C. Basilic   D. Median cubital

67. **What is the action of lumbricals on metacarpophalangeal joint?**
    A. Adduction   B. Flexion
    C. Abduction   D. Extension

68. **Clawhand deformity is due to damage of which nerve?**
    A. Ulnar   B. Median
    C. Radial   D. Axillary

69. **Which muscle flexes the distal interphalangeal joint?**
    A. Flexor digitorum superficialis
    B. Flexor digitorum profundus
    C. Palmar interossei
    D. Dorsal interossei

70. **What type of epiphysis is medial epicondyle of humerus?**
    A. Pressure   B. Traction
    C. Atavistic   D. Aberrant

71. What type of bursa is subscapular bursa?
A. Subcutaneous
B. Adventitious
C. Communicating
D. Non-communicating

72. Which one of the following is an ellipsoid variety of synovial joint?
A. Shoulder
B. Elbow
C. Wrist
D. 1st carpometacarpal

73. Which one of the following joints contain an articular disc?
A. Sternoclavicular
B. Shoulder
C. Elbow
D. Superior radioulnar

74. Which of the following muscles is supplied by two nerves?
A. Pronator teres
B. Flexor digitorum superficialis
C. Flexor pollocis longus
D. Flexor digitorum profundus

75. What type of cartilage covers the articular surface of sterno-clavicular joint?
A. Yellow elastic
B. White fibrous
C. Articular
D. None of the above

76. Which nerve supplies the adductor pollicis muscle?
A. Radial
B. Median
C. Superficial branch of ulnar
D. Deep branch of ulnar

77. What is the action of clavicular part of the deltoid muscle?
A. Flexion
B. Lateral rotation
C. Abduction
D. Extension

78. Each of the following has an attachment to scapula, EXCEPT:
A. Pectoralis major
B. Pectoralis minor
C. Biceps brachii
D. Triceps brachii

79. Following structures form the apex of the axilla, EXCEPT:
A. Clavicle
B. Coracoid process
C. Upper border of scapula
D. Outer border of first rib

80. Which muscle is called Boxer's muscle?
A. Trapezius
B. Serratus anterior
C. Pectoralis major
D. Latissimus dorsi

81. Muscles that can flex the elbow include all, EXCEPT:
A. Brachialis
B. Brachioradialis
C. Pronator teres
D. Anconeus

82. **Porter's tip deformity is seen in which one the following?**
   A. Klumpke's paralysis
   B. Radial nerve injury
   C. Ulnar nerve injury
   D. Erb's paralysis

83. **Which deformity is seen in injury to radial nerve?**
   A. Clawhand
   B. Ape thumb
   C. Winging of scapula
   D. Wrist drop

84. **Which deformity is seen in injury to long thoracic nerve?**
   A. Clawhand
   B. Ape thumb
   C. Winging of scapula
   D. Wrist drop

85. **Which deformity is seen in injury to ulnar nerve?**
   A. Clawhand
   B. Ape thumb
   C. Winging of scapula
   D. Wrist drop

86. **Lymphatics from the thumb directly drain into which lymph nodes?**
   A. Lateral
   B. Posterior
   C. Anterior
   D. Infraclavicular

87. **Which deformity is seen in injury to median nerve?**
   A. Claw hand
   B. Ape thumb
   C. Winging of scapula
   D. Wrist drop

88. **Which vein is most commonly used for blood collection and intravenous injection?**
   A. Basilic
   B. Cephalic
   C. Median cubital
   D. Axillary

89. **The intrinsic muscles of the hand are supplied by which spinal segments?**
   A. C5, C6
   B. C6, C7
   C. C7, C8
   D. C8, T1

90. **Brachialis is an example of which type of muscle?**
   A. Swing
   B. Spin.
   C. Spindle
   D. Shunt

91. **Which nerve may be damaged in dislocation of lunate bone?**
   A. Median
   B. Ulnar
   C. Radial
   D. None of the above

92. **Radial nerve passes through which one of the following?**
   A. Quadrangular space.
   B. Lower triangular space
   C. Upper triangular space
   D. Carpal tunnel

93. Inferior angle of the scapula lies at the level of which thoracic spine?
    A. 3   B. 5
    C. 6   D. 7

94. What is the dermatome of the middle finger?
    A. C6   B. C7
    C. C8   D. T1

95. Injury to which nerve causes regimental badge anaesthesia?
    A. Median   B. Musculocutaneous
    C. Axillary   D. Ulnar

96. Rupture of which tendon causes Popeye's deformity?
    A. Long head of triceps brachii
    B. Long head of biceps brachii
    C. Coracobrachialis
    D. Supraspinatus

97. Mallet finger deformity occurs due to rupture of which one of the following?
    A. Extensor expansion in the middle
    B. Extensor expansion in the terminal digit
    C. Flexor digitorum superficialis
    D. Extensor indicis tendon

98. Button hole finger deformity occurs due to rupture of which one of the following?
    A. Extensor expansion in the middle
    B. Extensor expansion in the terminal digit
    C. Flexor digitorum superficialis
    D. Extensor indicis tendon

99. All of the following nerves pass between two heads of the muscle, EXCEPT:
    A. Axillary   B. Median
    C. Musculocutaneus   D. Ulnar

100. Which is the site of injury to brachial plexus in Klumpke's paralysis?
    A. Upper trunk
    B. Middle trunk
    C. Lower trunk
    D. Lateral cord

101. Saturday night palsy deformity is due to damage of which nerve?

A. Ulnar

B. Median

C. Radial

D. Musculocutaneous

102. In fracture of surgical neck of humerus, which nerve is most likely to be injured?

A. Ulnar

B. Median

C. Radial

D. Axillary

103. In fracture of mid shaft of humerus, which nerve is most likely to be injured?

A. Ulnar

B. Median

C. Radial

D. Musculocutaneous

104. Which nerve roots are involved in Erb's paralysis?

A. C5, C6

B. C6, C7

C. C7, C8

D. C8, T1

105. Which nerve roots are involved in Klumpke's paralysis?

A. C5, C6

B. C6, C7

C. C7, C8

D. C8, T1

106. Through which one of the following axillary nerve passes?

A. Spiral groove

B. Upper triangular space

C. Lower triangular space

D. Quadrangular space

107. Which muscle connects the upper and lower limbs?

A. Trapezius

B. Psoas major

C. Latissimus dorsi

D. Serratus anterior

108. Superficial muscles of back of the thorax are supplied by which of the following nerve?

A. Ventral rami

B. Dorsal rami

C. Intercostal nerve

D. Dorsal root

109. Which vein is preferred for cardiac catheterization?

A. Median cubital

B. Basilic

C. Cephalic

D. Dorsal venous arch

110. Which nerve may be damaged in inferior dislocation of the shoulder joint?

A. Musculocutaneous

B. Long thoracic

C. Radial

D. Axillary

111. **In which one of the following bones flexor carpi radialis is inserted?**
    A. Scaphoid
    B. Trapezium
    C. Base of 1st metacarpal
    D. Base of 2nd metacarpal

112. **All of the following muscles are attached to the posterior border of ulna, EXCEPT:**
    A. Flexor carpi ulnaris
    B. Extersor carpi ulnaris
    C. Flexor digitorum superficialis
    D. Flexor digitorum profundus

113. **All of the following muscles are pierced by nerves, EXCEPT:**
    A. Supinator
    B. Pronator teres
    C. Coracobrachialis
    D. Brachialis

114. **Which nerve supplies medial two lumbricals of the hand?**
    A. Median
    B. Radial
    C. Superficial branch of ulnar
    D. Deep branch of ulnar

115. **What type of muscles is dorsal interossei of the hand?**
    A. Unipennate
    B. Bipennate
    C. Multipennate
    D. Circumpennate

116. **What type of muscles is palmar interossei of the hand?**
    A. Unipennate
    B. Bipennate
    C. Multipennate
    D. Circumpennate

117. **Which one of the following carpal bone is most commonly fractured?**
    A. Lunate
    B. Scaphoid
    C. Hammate
    D. Trapezium

118. **Which one of the following carpal bone is most commonly discolated?**
    A. Scaphoid
    B. Lunate
    C. Trapezium
    D. Hammate

119. **All of the following muscles take part in the lateral rotation of the scapula, EXCEPT:**
    A. Upper fibres of trapezius
    B. Middle fibres of trapezius
    C. Lower fibres of trapezius
    D. Lower 5 digitations of serratus anterior

120. **What type of muscles are medial two (3rd and 4th) lumbricals of the hand?**
   A. Unipennate
   B. Bipennate
   C. Multipennate
   D. Circumpennate

121. **What type of muscles are lateral two (1st and 2nd) lumbricals of the hand?**
   A. Unipennate
   B. Bipennate
   C. Multipennate
   D. Circumpennate

122. **Which nerve supplies lateral half of flexor digitorum profundus muscle?**
   A. Ulnar
   B. Median
   C. Radial
   D. Musculocutaneous

123. **Deep branches of the ulnar nerve supplies all of the following muscles, EXCEPT:**
   A. Palmaris brevis
   B. Adductor pollicis
   C. Palmar interossei
   D. Adbuctor digiti minimi

124. **Which muscle steadies the clavicle during movements of the pectoral girdle?**
   A. Deltoid
   B. Subclavius
   C. Pectoralis major
   D. Sternocleidomastoid

125. **Which part of the brachial plexus is the continuation of ventral ramus of the seventh cervical spinal nerve?**
   A. Upeer trunk
   B. Middle trunk
   C. Medial cord
   D. Lateral cord

126. **On which aspect interphalangeal joints in hand are devoid of capsule?**
   A. Medial
   B. Lateral
   C. Anterior
   D. Posterior

127. **All of the following connect the radius and ulna bones, EXCEPT:**
   A. Annular ligament
   B. Interosseous membrane
   C. Oblique cord
   D. Quadrate ligament

128. **All of the following are modifications of the deep fascia, EXCEPT:**
   A. Extensor retinaculum
   B. Extensor expansion
   C. Fibrous flexor sheath
   D. Palmar aponeurosis

129. Hammer thumb deformity is due to rupture of which one of the following tendons?
     A. Extensor pollicis longus   B. Flexor pollicis longus
     C. Extensor pollicis brevis   D. Flexor pollicis brevis

130. Coracohumeral ligament is a degenerated part of which one of the following?
     A. Short head of biceps brachii
     B. Pectoralis minor
     C. Subclavius
     D. Coracobrachialis

131. Oblique cord of the middle radioulnar joint is a degenerated part of which one of the following muscles?
     A. Flexor pollicis longus   B. Flexor digitorum profundus
     C. Pronator teres   D. Supinator

132. Median nerve supplies all of the following muscles of the thumb, EXCEPT:
     A. Abductor pollicis brevis
     B. Adductor pollicis
     C. Flexor pollicis brevis
     D. Opponens pollicis

133. A patient complains of loss of extension at the metacarpophalangeal joint. There is no wrist drop and extension of the interphalangel joints is normal. Which one of the following nerves is most likely to be involved?
     A. Median   B. Ulnar
     C. Radial   D. Posterior interosseous

134. Direct attachment of the pectoral girdle to the trunk is provided by all of the following muscles, EXCEPT:
     A. Pectoralis major   B. Pectoralis minor
     C. Trapezius   D. Subclavius

135. Which one of the following muscles provides indirect attachment of the pectoral girdle to the trunk?
     A. Pectoralis major   B. Pectoralis minor
     C. Trapezius   D. Subclavius

136. The scaphoid bone articulates all of the following, EXCEPT:
     A. Trapezium   B. Lunate
     C. Articular disc   D. Radius

137. A young man falls on his outstretched hand and complains of severe pain in his wrist in the anatomical snuff box. Which one of the following carpal bone is probably fractured?
   A. Trapezium
   B. Scaphoid
   C. Lunate
   D. Trapezoid

138. Lateral rotation of the shoulder joint is essential for full abduction of the arm. A blacksmith, therefore, needs a strong lateral rotator muscle such as:
   A. Supraspinatus
   B. Infraspinatus
   C. Teres major
   D. Latissimus dorsi

139. Which one of the following muscles can bring about extension, adduction and medial rotation of th shoulder joint?
   A. Deltoid
   B. Latissimus dorsi
   C. Subscapularis
   D. Teres minor

140. Which two muscles contract together in climbing?
   A. Latissimus dorsi and teres major
   B. Teres major and teres minor
   C. Teres major and pectoralis major
   D. Latissimus dorsi and pectoralis major

141. What is the continuation of the ventral ramus of the seventh cervical spinal nerve called?
   A. Upper trunk
   B. Middle trunk
   C. Medial cord
   D. Lateral cord

142. Which one of the following muscles helps a woman to keep her clutch bag tucked under her arm?
   A. Biceps brachii
   B. Deltoid
   C. Supraspinatus
   D. Coracobrachialis

143. Fracture of which one of the following bones is called boxer's fracture?
   A. Acromion process
   B. Scaphoid
   C. Hamate
   D. Head of 5th metacarpal

144. The biceps brachii is attached to all of the following, EXCEPT:
   A. Coracoid process
   B. Supraglenoid tubercle
   C. Shaft of humerus
   D. Radial tuberosity

145. All of the following muscles form posterior wall of the axilla, EXCEPT:
   A. Subscapularis
   B. Teres major
   C. Teres minor
   D. Latissimus dorsi

146. All of the following form boundaries of the triangle of auscultation, EXCEPT:

A. Medial border of scapula
B. Lateral border of trapezius
C. Upper border of teres major
D. Upper border of latissimus dorsi

147. All of the following form boundaries of the lumbar triangle of Petit, EXCEPT:

A. Quadratus lumborum
B. Iliac crest
C. Lateral border of latissimus dorsi
D. Posterior border of external oblique abdominis

148. Which one of the following nerves has a pseudoganglion?

A. Axillary
B. Long thoracic
C. Suprascapular
D. Nerve to teres minor

149. Up to which one of the following levels, ventral axial line extends?

A. Middle of arm
B. Proximal to elbow
C. Middle of forearm
D. Proximal to wrist

150. Up to which one of the following levels, dorsal axial line extends?

A. Middle of arm
B. Proximal to elbow
C. Middle of forearm
D. Proximal to wrist

151. All of the following muscles are medial rotators of the shoulder joint, EXCEPT:

A. Teres major
B. Teres minor
C. Pectoralis major
D. Latissimus dorsi

152. All of the following joints contain articular discs, EXCEPT:

A. Acromioclavicular
B. Sternoclavicular
C. Elbow
D. Wrist

153. All of the following muscles bing about retraction of the scapula, EXCEPT:

A. Rhomboideus major
B. Rhomboideus minor
C. Middle fibers of trapezius
D. Teres major

154. Which one of the following muscles, is flexor, adductor and medial rotator of the shoulder joint?

A. Pectoralis major
B. Pectoralis minor
C. Teres major
D. Infraspinatus

155. **Which one of the following muscles initiates abduction at the shoulder joint?**

   A. Deltoid
   B. Trapezius upper fibers
   C. Supraspinatus
   D. Trapezius middle fibers

156. **Which spinal nerve supplies the tip of the shoulder?**

   A. T2
   B. T3
   C. T4
   D. T5

157. **Which spinal segments supply the skin of the hand?**

   A. C4, 5, 6
   B. C5, 6, 7
   C. C6, 7, 8
   D. C7, 8, T1

158. **Which one of the following, would be the manifestation of the rupture of tendon of the supraspinatus?**

   A. Painful movements
   B. Flat shoulder
   C. Difficulty in initiation of abduction
   D. Difficult abduction after 90°

159. **Which branch of the axillar artery accompanies the long thoracic nerve?**

   A. Superior thoracic
   B. Subscapular
   C. Anterior circumflex humeral
   D. Lateral thoracic

160. **If entire greater tubercle of the humerus were torn away as a result of an injury, which of the following movements of shoulder would be affected?**

   A. Flexion and abduction
   B. Abudction and lateral rotation
   C. Flexion and medial rotation
   D. Extension and lateral rotation

161. **Which one of the following nerves gives rise to upper lateral cutaneous nerve of the arm?**

   A. Axillary
   B. Median
   C. Ulnar
   D. Radial

162. **Which one of the following structures may be injured by a deep laceration through the anatomical snuff box**

   A. Median nerve
   B. Radial nerve
   C. Radial artery
   D. Basilic vein

163. Which one of the following nerves gives rise to lower lateral cutaneous nerve of the arm?
    - A. Axillary
    - B. Median
    - C. Ulnar
    - D. Radial

164. Which one of the following nerves gives rise to posterior cutaneous nerve of the arm?
    - A. Axillary
    - B. Median
    - C. Ulnar
    - D. Radial

165. Which one of the following nerves gives rise to posterior cutaneous nerve of the forearm?
    - A. Axillary
    - B. Median
    - C. Ulnar
    - D. Radial

166. Which one of the following parts of the scapula forms the lateral most part palpable landmark on the shoulder?
    - A. Coracoid process
    - B. Glenoid cavity
    - C. Superior angle
    - D. Acromion process

167. Which one of the following nerves is called the eye of the hand?
    - A. Posterior interosseous
    - B. Median
    - C. Ulnar
    - D. Radial

168. Which one of the following nerves is called the musician's nerve?
    - A. Axillary
    - B. Median
    - C. Ulnar
    - D. Radial

169. Which one of the following nerves is called the labourer's nerve?
    - A. Axillary
    - B. Median
    - C. Ulnar
    - D. Radial

170. Which one of the following structures of the brachial plexus would most likely to be damaged in case of "winged scapula"?
    - A. Roots
    - B. Upper trunk
    - C. Middle trunk
    - D. Lateral cord

171. Integrity of which of the following muscles is tested by Formet's test?
    - A. Dorsal interossei
    - B. Palmar interossei
    - C. Lumbricals
    - D. Adductor pollicis

172. A patient has weakness flexing the metacarpophalangeal joint of the ring finger and is unable to adduct the same finger. Which of the following muscles is most likely paralysed?
    A. Flexor digitorum profundus
    B. Lumbricals
    C. Palmar interosseous
    D. Dorsal interosseous

173. A patient complains that she cannot flex her proximal interphalangeal joints. Which of the following muscles is most likely paralysed?
    A. Flexor digitorum profundus
    B. Flexor digitorum superficialis
    C. Palmar interossei
    D. Dorsal interossei

174. A man walks with a shoulder and arm injury after falling during motorbike riding. Examination indicates that he cannot adduct his arm because of paralysis of which of the following muscles?
    A. Supraspinatus   B. Infraspinatus
    C. Latissimus dorsi   D. Serratus anterior

175. A factory worker has his middle finger crushed in a machine. Which of the following muscles is most likely to retain its function?
    A. Palmar interosseous
    B. Dorsal interosseous
    C. Flexor digitorum profundus
    D. Lumbrical

176. A fracture of scaphoid bone is most likely accompanied by rupture of which of the following arteries?
    A. Anterior interosseous
    B. Princeps pollicis
    C. Deep palmar arterial arch
    D. Radial

177. A man involved in an automobile accident presents with arm that cannot abduct. His paralysis is caused by damage to which of the following nerves?
    A. Suprascapular and dorsal scapular
    B. Suprascapular and axillary
    C. Thoracodorsal and upper subscapular
    D. Axillary and musculocutaneous

178. A man complains of numbness on the medial side of the arm following a stab wound in the axilla, due to injury to the medial cutaneous nerve of the arm. In which of the following structures is the cell bodies of the damaged nerve invoved in numbness located?
    A. Anterior horn of spinal cord
    B. Posterior horn of spinal cord
    C. Lateral horn of spinal cord
    D. Dorsal root ganglion

179. Which one of the following pierces the interosseous membrane?
    A. Anterior interosseous nerve
    B. Anterior interosseous artery
    C. Posterior interosseous nerve
    D. Posterior interosseous artery

180. In cubital tunnel syndrome which of the following muscles is most likely to be paralysed?
    A. Flexor digitorum superficialis
    B. Proator teres
    C. Two medial lumbricals
    D. Opponens pollicis

181. A man complains of sensory loss, over the anterior and posterior surfaces of the medial third of the hand and medial one and half of fingers. Which of the following nerves is involved?
    A. Median
    B. Radial
    C. Musculocutaneous
    D. Ulnar

182. A woman is unable to hold a piece of paper between her index and middle fingers. Which of the following nerves was likely injured?
    A. Median
    B. Ulnar
    C. Radial
    D. Musculocutaneous

183. A blacksmith suffers a crush injury of his entire little finger. Which of the following muscles is most likely to be spared?
    A. Palmar interossei
    B. Dorsal interossei
    C. Lumbricals
    D. Extensor digitorum

184. Which of the following arteries is most likely to be damaged in fracture of the surgical neck of the humerus?
    A. Axillary
    B. Profunda brachii
    C. Circumflex scapular
    D. Posterior circumflex humeral

185. In an attempt to obtain a blood sample from the patient's median cubital vein, an intern inadvertently procures arterial blood. The blood most likely comes from which of the following arteries?

    A. Brachial
    B. Ulnar
    C. Radial
    D. Common interosseous

186. Which of the following arteries is most likely to be damaged in fracture of the shaft of the humerus?

    A. Brachial
    B. Profunda brachii
    C. Radial
    D. Posterior circumflex humeral

187. In an automobile accident a man has fracture of the shaft of the humerus. After this accident, supination is still possible through contraction of which of the following muscles?

    A. Supinator
    B. Biceps brachii
    C. Brachioradialis
    D. Anconeus

188. A boy has fracture of the surgical neck of the humerus. He has weakness in rotating his arm laterally. Which of the following muscles is paralysed?

    A. Teres major and teres minor
    B. Teres minor and deltoid
    C. Teres minor and infraspinatus
    D. Infraspinatus and deltoid

Interior Extremity

1. **Which one of the following drains into lateral group of superficial inguinal lymph nodes?**
   A. Lateral aspect of leg
   B. Gluteal region
   C. Dorsum of foot
   D. External genitalia

2. **Which nerve supplies the short head biceps femoris?**
   A. Anterior division of obturator
   B. Anterior division of femoral
   C. Common peroneal component of sciatic
   D. Tibial component of sciatic

3. **Which muscle extends the hip and laterally rotates the knee joint?**
   A. Adductor magnus.
   B. Semimembranosus.
   C. Biceps femoris
   D. Rectus femoris

4. **Which muscle connects the pelvic girdle to the upper limb?**
   A. External oblique abdominis
   B. Serratus anterior
   C. Latissimus dorsi
   D. Rectus abdominis

5. **In which quadrant of gluteal region should intermuscular injections be given to avoid damage to the sciatic nerve?**
   A. Upeer medial
   B. Upper lateral
   C. Lower lateral
   D. Lower medial

6. **Which muscle produces unlocking of the knee joint?**
   A. Quadratus femoris
   B. Biceps Femoris
   C. Popliteus.
   D. Quadriceps femoris

7. **Which bursa communicates with the knee joint?**
   A. Prepatellar
   B. Suprapatellar
   C. Superficial infrapatellar
   D. Deep infrapatellar

8. **Which muscle acts on both the knee and the ankle joints?**
   A. Soleus
   B. Gastrocnemius
   C. Flexor digitorum longus
   D. Peroneus longus

9. **Which nerve supplies plantar flexors of the foot?**
   A. Deep peroneal   B. Saphenous
   C. Tibial   D. Superficial peroneal

10. **Which nerve supplies lateral border of the foot?**
   A. Sural
   B. Saphenous
   C. Lateral cutaneous nerve of calf
   D. Superficial peroneal

11. **Which one of the following is the keystone of medial longitudinal arch of the foot?**
   A. Calcaneal tuberosity   B. Navicular tuberosity
   C. Base of 1st metatarsal D. Head of talus

12. **All of the following are antigravity muscles, EXCEPT:**
   A. Gluteus maximus.   B. Quadratus femoris
   C. Gastrocnemius   D. Soleus

13. **Morphologically, tibial collateral ligament represents degenerated tendons of which one of the following muscles?**
   A. Semitendinosus   B. Semimembranosus
   C. Adductor longus   D. Adductor magnus

14. **What type of joint is calcaneocuboid joint?**
   A. Plane   B. Saddle
   C. Ball and socket   D. Ellipsoid

15. **All of the following structures pass through porta pedis or tarsal tunnel, EXCEPT:**
   A. Tibialis posterior tendon B. Peroneal artery
   C. Tibial nerve   D. Posterior tibial artery

16. **What type of epiphysis is lower end of the femur?**
   A. Pressure   B. Traction
   C. Compound   D. Atavistic

17. **Which muscle passes through the lesser sciatic foramen?**
   A. Piriformis   B. Obturator externus
   C. Obturator internus   D. Quadratus femoris

18. **Distal part of which muscle is represented by plantar aponeurosis?**
   A. Soleus   B. Gastrocnemius
   C. Plantaris   D. Flexor digitorum longus

19. Sustentaculum tali is a part of which one of the following bones?

A. Talus
B. Calcaneus
C. Cuboid
D. Medial cuneiform

20. Which bursa is affected in clergyman's knee?

A. Infrapatellar
B. Semimembranous
C. Prepatellar
D. Suprapatellar

21. Which muscle is inserted in the navicular tuberosity?

A. Tibialis anterior
B. Peroneous longus
C. Tibialis posterior
D. Flexor hallucis longus

22. Saphenous nerve is a branch of which one of the following nerves?

A. Obturator
B. Tibial.
C. Femoral
D. Common peroneal

23. What type of joint is inferior tibiofibular joint?

A. Synchondrosis
B. Symphysis
C. Pivot
D. Syndesmosis

24. Which artery continues as the dorsalis pedis artery?

A. Anterior tibial
B. Posterior tibial
C. Peroneal
D. Lateral plantar

25. What is the root value of obturator nerve?

A. L1 L2
B. L4 L5 S1
C. L2 L3 L4
D. L4 L5 S1 S2 S3

26. Which nerve supplies the tensor fascia lata?

A. Sciatic
B. Inferior gluteal
C. Superior gluteal
D. Obturator

27. Football kick causes injury to which one of the following structures?

A. Lateral meniscus
B. Anterior cruciate ligament
C. Posterior cruciate ligament
D. Medial meniscus

28. Which muscle is the evertor of the foot?

A. Peroneus longus
B. Tibialis anterior
C. Tibialis posterior
D. Flexor hallucis longus

29. **Which muscle locks the knee joint?**
    A. Popliteus
    B. Gastrocnemius.
    C. Quadratus femoris
    D. Quadriceps femoris

30. **Which bone is devoid of muscular attachments?**
    A. Cuboid
    B. Talus
    C. Navicular
    D. Medial cuneiform

31. **Positive Trendelenburg's sign could result from paralysis of which muscle?**
    A. Gluteus medius
    B. Gluteus maximus
    C. Psoas major
    D. Adductor magnus

32. **Which nerve supplies the dorsiflexors of the foot?**
    A. Tibial
    B. Saphenous
    C. Deep peroneal
    D. Superficial peroneal

33. **Which bursa is called housemaid's bursa?**
    A. Suprapatellar
    B. Prepatellar
    C. Subcutaneous infrapatellar
    D. Deep infrapatellar

34. **Which structure is innervated by the posterior division of obturator nerve?**
    A. Hip joint
    B. Knee joint
    C. Adductor longus
    D. Pectineus

35. **All of the following bones take part in the formation of lateral longitudinal arch of the foot, EXCEPT:**
    A. Calcaneus
    B. Cuboid
    C. Navicular
    D. Fifth metatarsal

36. **In sitting position the weight of the body is supported by which structure?**
    A. Pubic arch
    B. Ischial tuberosity
    C. Ramus of the ischium
    D. Body of pubis

37. **Which muscle forms the superolateral boundary of popliteal fossa?**
    A. Vastus lateralis
    B. Plantaris
    C. Biceps femoris
    D. Lateral head of gastrocnemius

38. **Which muscle is inserted into the iliotibial tract?**
    A. Gluteus minimus
    B. Gluteus medius
    C. Gluteus maximus
    D. Quadratus femoris

39. Abduction and adduction of the fore foot occurs at which joint?

A. Subtalar   B. Midtarsal
C. Inferior tibiofibular   D. Ankle

40. Which is the most stable position of the foot?

A. Inversion   B. Plantar flexion
C. Eversion   D. Dorsiflexion

41. In to which lymph nodes lymphatics drain from heel and lateral part of foot?

A. Superficial inguinal   B. Deep inguinal
C. External iliac   D. Popliteal

42. Which muscle connects vertebral column to the lower limb?

A. Biceps femoris   B. Quadratus lumborum
C. Rectus femoris   D. Psoas major

43. Superior gluteal nerve supplies all of the following muscles, EXCEPT:

A. Gluteus maximus   B. Gluteus medius
C. Gluteus minimus   D. Tensor fascia lata

44. What type of muscle is tibialis anterior?

A. Bipennate   B. Fusiform
C. Strap like   D. Circumpennate

45. Adductor canal contains all of the following, EXCEPT:

A. Femoral artery
B. Nerve to vastus medialis
C. Femoral nerve
D. Saphenous nerve

46. Tibial part of sciatic nerve supplies all of the following muscles EXCEPT

A. Short head of biceps femoris
B. Semitendinosus
C. Semimembranosus
D. Ischial head of adductor magnus

47. From which structure sartorius muscle takes origin?

A. Pectinate line
B. Anterior superior iliac spine
C. Anterior inferior iliac spine
D. Ischial tuberosity

48. All of the following structures pass through the lesser sciatic foramen, EXCEPT:
A. Obturator internus tendon
B. Pudendal nerve
C. Internal pudendal vessels
D. Superior gluteal nerve

49. What is the action of quadratus femoris at the hip joint?
A. Extension
B. Flexion
C. Lateral rotation
D. Medial rotation

50. Which artery is present in the adductor canal?
A. Profunda femoris
B. Femoral
C. Obturator
D. Popliteal

51. Which muscle froms the superomedial boundary of the popliteal fossa?
A. Vastus medialis
B. Popliteus
C. Semitendinosus
D. Medial head of gastrocnemius

52. Femoral nerve supplies all of the following muscles, EXCEPT:
A. Sartorius
B. Rectus femoris
C. Tensor fascia lata
D. Articularis genu

53. Which muscle passes through to greater sciatic foramen?
A. Obturator internus
B. Obturator externus
C. Piriformis
D. Quadratus femoris

54. The companion artery of the sciatic nerve (arteria nervi ischiadica) is branch of which artery?
A. Internal pudendal
B. Profunda femoris
C. Superior gluteal
D. Inferior gluteal

55. What type of talipes deformity is seen in injury to tibial nerve?
A. Calcaneovarus
B. Calcaneovalgus
C. Equinovarus
D. Equinovalgus

56. Gluteal region communicates with which of the following structure?
A. Pelvic cavity
B. Ischio-rectal fossa
C. Posterior compartment of thigh
D. All of the above

57. The insertion of the adductor magnus muscle on linea aspera is interrupted by how many osseo-aponeurotic openings?
    A. Two
    B. Three
    C. Four
    D. Five

58. All of the following bones take a part in the formation of medial longitudinal arch of the foot, EXCEPT:
    A. Calcaneus
    B. Cuboid
    C. Navicular
    D. Medial cuneiform

59. What type of joint is superior tibofibular joint?
    A. Syndesmosis
    B. Plane synovial
    C. Symphysis
    D. Synchondrosis

60. What type of joint is middle tibiofibular joint?
    A. Syndesmosis
    B. Plane synovial
    C. Symphysis
    D. Synchondrosis

61. What type of joint is talocalcaneonavicular joint?
    A. Plane
    B. Saddle
    C. Ball and socket
    D. Ellipsoid

62. What type of joint is femoropatellar joint?
    A. Plane
    B. Saddle
    C. Ball and socket
    D. Ellipsoid

63. Morphologically fibular collateral ligament represents degenerated tendon of which one of the following muscles?
    A. Biceps femoris
    B. Peroneus longus
    C. Adductor magnus
    D. Lateral head of gastrocnemius

64. Morphologically, long plantar ligament represents degenerated tendon of which one of the following muscles?
    A. Gastrocnemius
    B. Plantaris
    C. Soleus
    D. Peroneus brevis

65. Morphologically plantar aponeurosis represents degenerated tendon of which one of the following muscles?
    A. Gastrocnemius
    B. Plantaris
    C. Soleus
    D. Peroneus brevis

66. Morphologically, oblique popliteal ligament represents degenerated tendon of which one of the following muscles?
    A. Semitendinosus
    B. Semimembranosus
    C. Gracilis
    D. Biceps femoris

67. Flexor digitorum brevis is detached part of which muscle?

A. Gastrocnemius   B. Plantaris

C. Soleus   D. Plopliteus

68. All of the following are hamstring muscles, EXCEPT:

A. Short head of biceps femoris

B. Semitendinosus

C. Semimembranosus

D. Ischial head of adductor

69. Anterior division of obturator nerve supplies all of the following muscles, EXCEPT:

A. Adductor longus   B. Adductor brevis

C. Adductor magnus   D. Pectineus

70. What is the position of line of gravity in relation to the hip joint?

A. Medial   B. Lateral

C. Anterior   D. Posterior

71. What is the position of line of gravity in relation to the knee joint?

A. Medial   B. Lateral

C. Anterior   D. Posterior

72. What is the position of line of gravity in relation to the ankle joint?

A. Medial   B. Lateral

C. Anterior   D. Posterior

73. All of the structures pass through saphenous opening, EXCEPT:

A. Great saphenous vein

B. Superficial external pudendal artery

C. Superficial epigastric artery

D. Superficial circumflex iliac artery

74. Which structure is present in the femoral canal?

A. Cloquet's lymph node

B. Femoral artery

C. Femoral vein

D. Femoral branch of genitofemoral nerve

75. Which type of gait is seen in unilateral paralysis of gluteus medius muscle?

A. Lurching   B. Waddling

C. Scissors   D. Propulsion

76. **Which type of gait is seen in bilateral paralysis of gluteus medius muscle?**
    A. Lurching
    B. Waddling
    C. Scissors
    D. Propulsion

77. **In paralysis of which muscle patient cannot stand up from sitting position without support?**
    A. Quadratus femoris
    B. Gluteus maximus
    C. Gluteus medius
    D. Gastrocnemius

78. **Rider's bone develops in the tendinous origin of which muscle?**
    A. Sartorius
    B. Adductor longus
    C. Obturator externus
    D. Gracilis

79. **Anserine bursa lies between insertions of all the following muscles, EXCEPT:**
    A. Semitendinosus
    B. Semimembranosus
    C. Gracilis
    D. Sartorius

80. **All the following muscles are called Guy rope muscles, EXCEPT:**
    A. Semitendinosus
    B. Semimembranosus
    C. Gracilis
    D. Sartorius

81. **All the following muscles are supplied by obturator nerve, EXCEPT:**
    A. Obturator internus
    B. Obturator externus
    C. Gracilis
    D. Pectineus

82. **During locking of the knee joint which ligament acts as a vertical axis around which medial condyle of femur rotates?**
    A. Anterior cruciate
    B. Posterior cruciate
    C. Fibular collateral
    D. Tibial collateral

83. **Paralysis which muscles will result in high stepping gait?**
    A. Evertors
    B. Invertors
    C. Dorsi flexors
    D. Plantar flexors

84. **Which one of the following structures acts as intersegmental tie for maintaining medial longitudinal arch of the foot?**
    A. Long plantar ligament
    B. Spring ligament
    C. Plantar aponeurosis
    D. Deep transverse ligament

85. Which one of the following structures acts as intersegmental tie for maintaining lateral longitudinal arch of the foot?

    A. Long plantar ligament   B. Spring ligament

    C. Plantar aponeurosis   D. Deep transverse ligament

86. Which one of the following structures acts as intersegmental tie for maintaining transverse arch of the foot?

    A. Long plantar ligament   B. Spring ligament

    C. Plantar aponeurosis   D. Deep transverse ligament

87. All of the following structures act as tie beam to maintain both medial and lateral longitudinal arches of the foot, EXCEPT:

    A. Plantar aponeurosis   B. Flexor digitorum brevis

    C. Flexor digitorum longus   D. Adductor hallucis

88. What type of telipes deformity is seen in injury to common peroneal nerve?

    A. Calcaneovarus   B. Calcaneovalgus

    C. Equinovarus   D. Equinovalgus

89. Which artery joins the lateral plantar artery to from plantar arch?

    A. Medial plantar   B. Peroneal

    C. Anterior tibial   D. Dorsalis pedis

90. Which fascia forms anterior wall of the femoral sheath?

    A. Iliaca   B. Transversalis

    C. Cribriform   D. Lata

91. Which fascia forms posterior wall of the femoral sheath?

    A. Cribriform   B. Lata

    C. Iliaca   D. Transversalis

92. What is the course of the an enlarging femoral hernial sac?

    A. Downwards, backwards, upwards

    B. Downwards, forwards, medially

    C. Downwards, forwards, laterally

    D. Downwards forwards, upwards

93. All of the following are branches of femoral artery, EXCEPT:

    A. Superficial external pudendal

    B. Deep external pudendal

    C. Superficial circumflex iliac

    D. Superior epigastric

94. **What is the relationship of the saphenous opening to the pubic tubercle?**
    A. Above and medial
    B. Above and lateral
    C. Below and medial
    D. Below and lateral

95. **All of the following components of the quadriceps femoris muscle are attached the femur, EXCEPT:**
    A. Vastus medialis
    B. Rectus femoris
    C. Articularis genu
    D. Vastus lateralis

96. **The nutrient artery to the fibula is a branch of which artery?**
    A. Anterior tibial
    B. Posterior tibial
    C. Popliteal
    D. Peroneal

97. **The nutrient artery to the tibia is a branch of which artery?**
    A. Anterior tibial
    B. Posterior tibial
    C. Popliteal
    D. Peroneal

98. **Injury to which nerve causes foot drop?**
    A. Tibial
    B. Femoral
    C. Obturator
    D. Common peroneal

99. **Which muscle is called tailor's muscle?**
    A. Gluteus maximus
    B. Quadriceps femoris
    C. Semitendinosus
    D. Sartorius

100. **In case of block of femoral artery at its commencement which artery will supply the lower limb?**
    A. Superior gluteal
    B. Inferior gluteal
    C. Obturator
    D. Inferior epigastic

101. **Which ligament is pierced by middle genicular nerve?**
    A. Tibial collateral
    B. Fibular collateral
    C. Ligamentum pattellae
    D. Oblique popliteal

102. **In fracture neck femur the distal fragment is rotated laterally due to contraction of all of the following muscles, EXCEPT:**
    A. Gluteus maximus
    B. Gluteus medius
    C. Psoas major
    D. Piriformis

103. **Neck of the fibula is related to which nerve?**
    A. Superficial peroneal
    B. Common peroneal
    C. Deep peroneal
    D. Tibial

104. Which one of the following muscles is called peripheral heart?

A. Gluteus maximus   B. Popliteus

C. Soleus   D. Plantaris

105. Which muscle is supplied by common peroneal component of the sciatic nerve?

A. Semitendinosus

B. Short head of biceps femoris

C. Long head of biceps femoris

D. Semimembranosus

106. At which joint movements of inversion and eversion take place?

A. Subtalar   B. Transverse tarsal

C. Talocalcaneonavicular   D. All of the above

107. Inferior gluteal nerve supplies which muscle/muscles?

A. Gluteus maximus   B. Gluteus medius

C. Gluteus minimus   D. All of the above

108. In fracture neck femur the distal fragment is pulled upwards and shortened due to contraction of all of the following muscles, EXCEPT:

A. Rectus femoris   B. Adductors

C. Hamstrings   D. Quadratus femoris

109. Which nerve may be damaged in posterior dislocation of the hip joint?

A. Obturator   B. Sciatic

C. Femoral   D. Pudendal

110. Tibialis posterior is inserted to all of the following, EXCEPT:

A. Medial cuneiform   B. Navicular

C. First metatarsal   D. 3rd metatarsal

111. Which ligament is rendered taut in inversion?

A. Cervical   B. Deltoid

C. Spring   D. Long plantar

112. Sacrotuberous ligament is a degenerated part of which muscle?

A. Biceps femoris   B. Semitendinosus

C. Semimembranosus   D. Adductor longus

113. Tears of the all of the following structures are seen in 'unhappy triad' of the knee joint, EXCEPT:
    A. Medial meniscus   B. Lateral meniscus
    C. Anterior cruciate ligament D. Tibial collateral ligament

114. Avascular necrosis of head of femur is maximum in which one of the fractures of the femur?
    A. Subcapital   B. Cervical
    C. Trochanteric   D. Mid shaft

115. What type of muscle is 1st lumbrical of the foot?
    A. Unipennate   B. Bipennate
    C. Multipennate   D. Circumpennate

116. What type of muscles are lateral three lumbricals of the foot?
    A. Unipennate   B. Bipennate
    C. Multipennate   D. Circumpennate

117. What type of muscles are dorsal interossei of the foot?
    A. Unipennate   B. Bipennate
    C. Multipennate   D. Circumpennate

118. What type of muscles are plantar interossei of the foot?
    A. Unipennate   B. Bipennate
    C. Multipennate   D. Circumpennate

119. In to which one of the following flexor accessorius muscle is inserted?
    A. Medial cuneiform   B. Navicular
    C. Flexor digitorum brevis   D. Flexor digitorum longus

120. The accumulated blood in the synovial cavity of knee joint can be removed through which one of the following bursae?
    A. Prepatellar   B. Superficial infrapatellar
    C. Deep infrapatellar   D. Suprapatellar

121. Which muscle enables you to arise out of chair and straighten your trunk over your lower extremities?
    A. Gluteus maximus   B. Gluteus medius
    C. Psoas major   D. Adductor magnus

122. A child falls on a spike injuring the upper lateral margin of the popliteal fossa. Which one of the following nerves is liable to injury?
    A. Tibial   B. Common peroneal
    C. Femoral   D. Sciatic

123. If the tendocalceneus is severed as a punishment to a convicted prisoner, he would be still able to flex his ankle by which one of the following muscles?

A. Peroneus tertius   B. Tibialis anterior
C. Sloeus   D. Flexor hallusis longus

124. Which one of the following ligaments of the knee joint, is maximally taut while walking downhill?

A. Medial collateral   B. Lateral collateral
C. Anterior cruciate   D. Posterior cruciate

125. Which one of the following ligaments prevents the forward displacement of the femur on the tibia at the knee joint?

A. Anterior cruciate   B. Posterior cruciate
C. Transverse   D. Patellar

126. Which one of the following ligaments is taut during flexion of the knee joint?

A. Anterior cruciate   B. Posterior cruciate
C. Transverse   D. Patellar

127. Which one of the following ligaments is taut during extension of the knee joint?

A. Anterior cruciate   B. Posterior cruciate
C. Transverse   D. Patellar

128. Which one of the following ligaments prevents the backward displacement of the femur on the tibia at the knee joint?

A. Anterior cruciate   B. Posterior cruciate
C. Transverse   D. Patellar

129. Fatty pads (haversian pads) are found in all of the following joints, EXCEPT:

A. Hip   B. Knee
C. Ankle   D. Talocalcaneonavicular

130. Which muscle extends the hip joint and flexes the knee joint?

A. Sartorius
B. Rectus femoris
C. Long head of biceps femoris
D. Short head of biceps femoris

131. Which muscle flexes the hip joint and extends the knee joint?

A. Sartorius   B. Rectus femoris
C. Gracilis   D. Long head of biceps femoris

132. Plantar arch lies between which layers of the sole?
- A. First and second
- B. Second and third
- C. Third and fourth
- D. Deep to fourth

133. In to which one of the following flexor accessories is inserted?
- A. Base of the distal phalanx
- B. Base of the proximal phalanx
- C. Flexor digitorum brevis
- D. Flexor digitorum longus

134. All of the following are muscle of the first layer of the sole, EXCEPT:
- A. Flexor digitorum brevis
- B. Abductor hallucis
- C. Abductor digiti minimi
- D. Adductor hallucis

135. All of the following are muscle of the second layer of the sole, EXCEPT:
- A. Tendon of flexor hallucis longus
- B. Flexor digitorum brevis
- C. Lumbricals
- D. Flexor accessories

136. All of the following are muscle of the third layer of the sole, EXCEPT:
- A. Flexor hallucis brevis
- B. Flexor digiti minimi brevis
- C. Abductor hallucis
- D. Adductor hallucis

137. All of the following are branches of the dorsalis pedis artery, EXCEPT:
- A. Arcuate
- B. Medial tarsal
- C. Lateral tarsal
- D. Medial plantar

138. Which one of the following artery is a branch of the posterior tibial artery?
- A. Arcuate
- B. Medial tarsal
- C. Lateral tarsal
- D. Medial plantar

139. In which one of the following movements of the knee joint, medial strip on the posterior surface of the patella comes in contact with femur?
- A. Slight flexion
- B. Mid flexion
- C. Full flexion
- D. Extension

140. Which part of ischial tuberosity supports the body weight in sitting?
- A. Upper superolateral
- B. Upper inferomedial
- C. Lower outer
- D. Lower inner

141. **All of the following are attached to the greater trochanter of the femur, EXCEPT:**
    A. Gluteus maximus
    B. Gluteus medius
    C. Obturator internus
    D. Obturator externus

142. **Tendon of which muscle occupies groove on the lower surface of the sustentaculum tali of the calcaneum?**
    A. Flexor hallucis longus
    B. Flexor digitorum longus
    C. Flexor hallucis brevis
    D. Tibialis posterior

143. **Which one of the following tarsal bones has a groove on the plantar surface for the passage of tendon of peroneus longus?**
    A. Calcaneum
    B. Cuboid
    C. Navicular
    D. Lateral cuneiform

144. **Which part of the thigh is the preferred site to give intra-muscular injections in children?**
    A. Anteromedial
    B. Anterolateral
    C. Posteromedial
    D. Posterolateral

145. **Which one of the following is a hybrid muscle?**
    A. Adductor brevis
    B. Adductor longus
    C. Adductor magnus
    D. Sartorius

146. **Tibialis posterior is inserted into all of the following, EXCEPT:**
    A. Base of 1st metatarsal
    B. Base of 2nd metatarsal
    C. Base of 3rd metatarsal
    D. Cuboid

147. **All of the following muscles are supplied by medial plantar nerve, EXCEPT:**
    A. Flexor digitorum brevis
    B. Flexor hallucis brevis
    C. Adductor hallucis
    D. Abductor hallucis

148. **How many valves are present in long saphenous vein?**
    A. 5–6
    B. 10–20
    C. 24–25
    D. 28–30

149. **How many degrees is the neck shaft angle of femur in adults?**
    A. 100
    B. 110
    C. 125
    D. 135

150. **All of the following muscles are attached to the calcaneus, EXCEPT:**
    A. Flexor digitorum accessorius
    B. Abductor hallucis

C. Extensor digitorum brevis

D. Adductor hallucis

151. Which one of the following muscls dorsiflexes the foot at the ankle joint?

A. Tibialis anterior

B. Peroneus longus

C. Extensor digitorum brevis

D. Extensor hallucis longus

152. The superficial circumflex iliac artery usually anastomoses with which of the following arteries?

A. Ascending branch of lateral circumflex femoral

B. Deep circumflex iliac

C. Deep branch of superior gluteal

D. All of the above

153. All of the following arteries take part in the trochanteric anastomoses, EXCEPT:

A. Branch of superior gluteal

B. Branch of inferior gluteal

C. Ascending branch of lateral circumflex

D. Transverse branch of medial circumflex femoral

154. All of the following arteries take part in the cruciate anastomoses, EXCEPT:

A. Branch of superior gluteal

B. Ascending branch of 1st perforaring

C. Transverse branch of lateral circumflex

D. Transverse branch of medial circumflex femoral femoral

155. The longitudinal anastomoses on the back of the thigh is formed by branches of all of the following arteries, EXCEPT:

A. Internal iliac

B. Femoral

C. Popliteal

D. Anterior tibial

156. Origin of which one of the following muscles is intracapsular?

A. Plantaris

B. Popliteus

C. Medial head of gastrocnemius

D. Lateral head of gastrocnemius

157. Which spinal nerves supply the skin of the sole?
    A. L2, 3   B. L3,4
    C. L4,5   D. L5, S1

158. Deep circumflex iliac artery is a branch of which one of the following arteries?
    A. Internal iliac   B. External iliac
    C. Femoral   D. Inferior epigastric

159. How many centimeters anterior to the medial malleolus, great saphenous vein can be exposed?
    A. 1   B. 1.5
    C. 2.5   D. 3.5

160. Which one of the following is the longest muscle?
    A. Adductor longus
    B. Peroneus longus
    C. Flexor digitorum longus
    D. Sartorius

161. Through which one of the following, profunda femoris artery leaves the femoral triangle?
    A. Apex of the femoral triangle
    B. Behind sartorius
    C. Between pectineus and adductor longus
    D. Between pectineus and psoas major

162. In which one of the following, femoral branch of the genito-femoral nerve is located?
    A. Inguinal canal
    B. Femoral canal
    C. Medial compartment of femoral sheath
    D. Lateral compartment of femoral sheath

163. To which one of the following menisci, meniscofemoral ligaments are attached?
    A. Anterior horn of medial   B. Posterior horn of medial
    C. Anterior horn of lateral   D. Posterior horn of lateral

164. Obturator artery is a branch of which one of the following arteries?
    A. Common iliac
    B. External iliac
    C. Anterior division of internal iliac
    D. Posterior division of internal iliac

165. **Violent inversion of foot, results in avulsion of which one of the following tendons?**
     A. Peroneus longus   B. Peroneus brevis
     C. Peroneus tertius   D. Tibialis posterior

166. **Which one of the following nerves is tested, when a doctor pinches the skin between the big toe and second toe?**
     A. Saphenous   B. Sural
     C. Superficial peroneal   D. Deep peroneal

167. **A patient with deep knife wound in the buttock walks with a waddling gait. Which of the following nerves is damaged?**
     A. Obturator   B. Nerve to obturator internus
     C. Superior gluteal   D. Inferior gluteal

168. **A rupture of the ligamentum teres capitis femoris may lead to damage to a branch of which of the following arteries?**
     A. Superior gluteal   B. Inferior gluteal
     C. Obturator   D. Medial circumflex femoral

169. **Fracture of neck of the femur results in avascular necrosis of the femoral head, probably resulting from the lack of blood supply from which of the following arteries?**
     A. Superior gluteal
     B. Inferior gluteal
     C. Medial circumflex femoral
     D. Lateral circumflex femoral

170. **If the acetabulum is fractured at its posterosuperior margin by dislocation of the hip joint, which of the following bones could be involved?**
     A. Ilium   B. Ischium
     C. Pubis   D. Sacrum

171. **A man sustains a fracture of the groove on the undersurface of the susterntaculum tali of the calcaneus bone. Which of the following muscle tendon is most likely torn?**
     A. Flexor hallucis brevis   B. Flexor hallucis longus
     C. Flexor digitorum brevis D. Flexor digitorum longus

172. **A man sustains a fracture of the groove on the lower surface of the cuboid bone. Which of the following muscle tendon is most likely torn?**
     A. Flexor hallucis longus   B. Tibialis anterior
     C. Peroneus brevis   D. Peroneus longus

173. A patient experiences weakness in dorsiflexing and inverting the foot. Which of the following muscle is damaged?

    A. Peroneus longus   B. Peroneus brevis

    C. Peroneus tertius   D. Tibialis anterior

174. If obturator nerve is damaged which one of the following muscles is completely paralysed?

    A. Adductor magnus   B. Adductor longus

    C. Biceps femoris   D. Pectineus

175. A patient presents with a thrombosis in the popliteal vein. This thrombosis most likely causes reduction of blood flow in which of the following veins?

    A. Long saphenous   B. Short saphenous

    C. Femoral   D. Anterior tibial

Thorax

1. What is the dermatome at the level of sternal angle?
    A. T1   B. T 2
    C. T 3   D. T4

2. Which vessels supply oxygenated blood to the lungs?
    A. Pulmonary arteries   B. Pulmonary veins
    C. Coronary arteries   D. Bronchial arteries

3. Which is the most anterior structure at the root of the lung?
    A. Pulmonary artery   B. Superior pulmonary vein
    C. Primary bronchus.   D. Bronchial artery

4. Each bronchopulmonary segment is aerated by which one of the following?
    A. Secondary bronchus   B. Tertiary bronchus
    C. Terminal bronchiole   D. Respiratory bronchiole

5. All of the following structures are related to the medial surface of right lung, EXCEPT:
    A. Superoir vena cava   B. Oesophagus
    C. Thoracic duct   D. Trachea

6. The right atrium receives blood from each of the following, EXCEPT:
    A. Pulmonary vein   B. Coronary sinus
    B. Inferior vena cava   D. Superior vena cava

7. Which is the longest rib?
    A. Seventh   B. Eight
    C. Ninth   D. Tenth

8. All of the following are branches of the arch of the aorta, EXCEPT:
    A. Left common carotid   B. Left subclavian
    C. Brachiocephalic   D. Right subclavian

9. Which diameter of the thorax is increased by the bucket handle movements of the ribs?
   A. Transverse
   B. Antero-posterior
   C. Vertical
   D. Oblique

10. Which is the most superior structure at the root of the left lung?
    A. Pulmonary artery
    B. Superior pulmonary vein
    C. Primary bronchus
    D. Bronchial artery

11. Crista terminalis is seen in the interior of which chamber of the heart?
    A. Left atrium
    B. Right atrium
    C. Left ventricle
    D. Right ventricle

12. Transverse sinus lies between which two layers of pericardium?
    A. Fibrous and parietal
    B. Parietal and visceral
    C. Parietal and parietal
    D. Visceral and visceral

13. All of the following are contents of the posterior mediastinum, EXCEPT:
    A. Oesophagus
    B. Trachea
    C. Thoracic duct
    D. Azygos vein

14. Which is the most oblique rib?
    A. Seventh
    B. Eighth
    C. Nineth
    D. Tenth

15. The base of the heart is formed by which of the following?
    A. Right atrium
    B. Left atrium
    C. Right and left atrium
    D. Right and left ventricles

16. At which thoracic vertebral level trachea divides?
    A. 1
    B. 2
    C. 4
    D. 6

17. Which chamber of the heart when enlarged will compress the oesophagus?
    A. Right atrium
    B. Left atrium
    C. Right ventricle
    D. Left ventricle

18. The sympathetic nerve supply to the heart is derived from which of the following spinal segments?
    A. C 8 to T 2
    B. T2 to T5
    C. T4 to T6
    D. T5 to T9

19. Oblique sinus lies between which two layers of pericardium?
- A. Visceral and visceral
- B. Visceral and parietal
- C. Parietal and fibrous
- D. Parietal and parietal

20. What type of joint is first chondrosternal joint?
- A. Synovial
- B. Fibrous
- C. Primary cartilaginous
- D. Secondary cartilaginous

21. Thoracic duct crosses from right side to the left at the level of which thoracic vertebra?
- A. 3
- B. 5
- C. 6
- D. 7

22. Which diameter of the thorax is increased by pump handle movements of ribs?
- A. Vertical
- B. Transverse
- C. Anteroposterior
- D. Oblique

23. Which is the typical intercostal space?
- A. Second
- B. Fifth
- C. Seventh
- D. Ninth

24. What type of synovial joint is costovertebral joint?
- A. Hinge
- B. Plane
- C. Ellipsoid
- D. Saddle

25. Anterior intercostal arteries are branches of which artery?
- A. Internal thoracic
- B. Posterior intercostal
- C. Costocervical trunk
- D. Superior epigastric

26. Internal thoracic artery is branch of which artery?
- A. Arch of aorta
- B. Subclavian artery
- C. Axillary artery
- D. Brachiocephalic trunk

27. What is the location of sinoatrial node?
- A. Septal cusp of tricuspid valve
- B. The opening of coronary sinus
- C. Limbus fossa ovalis
- D. Upper end of crista terminalis

28. Which nerve supplies fibrous pericardium?
- A. Vagus
- B. Phrenic
- C. Sympathetic
- D. Intercostal

29. To which structure superficial cardiac plexus is related?
- A. Below arch of the aorta
- B. Right coronary artery
- C. Pulmonary trunk
- D. Superior vena cava

30. To which structure deep cardiac plexus is related?
   A. Myocardium
   B. Oblique sinus
   C. Termination of superior vena cava
   D. Bifurcation of trachea

31. Which cardiac vein accompanies the anterior interventricular branch of coronary artery?
   A. Anterior   B. Great
   C. Middle   D. Small

32. Which cardiac vein accompanies the posterior interventricular branch of right coronary artery?
   A. Anterior   B. Great
   C. Middle   D. Small

33. Artery supplying the anterior part of interventricular septum is a branch of which artery?
   A. Circumflex   B. Right coronary
   C. Left coronary   D. Marginal branch of right

34. Which thoracic sympathetic ganglia contribute to greater splanchnic nerve?
   A. 2 to 4   B. 5 to 9
   C. 8 to 10   D. 11 and 12

35. Which nerves supply costal part of parietal pleura?
   A. Phrenic   B. Vagus
   C. Sympathetic   D. Intercostal

36. All of the following structures pass through thoracic inlet, EXCEPT:
   A. Trachea   B. Oesophagus
   C. Supeior vena cava   D. Vagus nerve

37. Right bronchial artery is a brach of which artery?
   A. Ascending aorta
   B. Arch of the aorta
   C. Descending aorta
   D. Right third posterior intercostal

38. Azygos vein opens into which vein?
   A. Superior vena cava   B. Hemiazygos
   C. Accessory hemiazygos   D. Inferior vena cava

39. Which artery of the heart is responsible for cardiac dominance?
    A. Anterior interventricular   B. Posterior interventricular
    C. Marginal   D. Infundibular

40. Following cardiac veins are the tributaries of coronary sinus, EXCEPT:
    A. Great   B. Middle
    C. Anterior   D. Small

41. What type of joint is manubriosternal joint?
    A. Primary cartilaginous   B. Secondary cartilaginous
    C. Syndesmosis   D. Plane synovial

42. All of the following structures are present in the posterior mediastinum, EXCEPT:
    A. Oesophagus   B. Trachea
    C. Descending thoracic aorta   D. Azygos vein

43. Artery supplying the posterior part of interventricular septum is a branch of which artery?
    A. Circumflex   B. Right coronary
    C. Left coronary   D. Marginal branch of right

44. All of the following structures are related to mediastinal surface of the left lung, EXCEPT:
    A. Pulmonary trunk   B. Arch of aorta
    C. Azygos vein   D. Left brachiocephalic vein

45. Left bronchial arteries are branches of which artery?
    A. Left 3rd posterior intercostal
    B. Left 5th posterior intercostal
    C. Descending thoracic aorta
    D. Brachiocephalic

46. All of the following structures are related to neck of the first rib, EXCEPT:
    A. Sympathetic chain   B. First posterior intercostal vein
    C. First thoracic nerve   D. Subclavian vein

47. Which one of the following is an example of atypical intercostal nerve?
    A. Fourth   B. Fifth
    C. Sixth   D. Seventh

48. Central part of parietal layer of diaphragmatic pleura is supplied by which nerve?
    A. Intercostal
    B. Subcostal
    C. Phrenic
    D. Vagus

49. Coronary arteries are branches of which artery?
    A. Ascending aorta
    B. Arch of aorta
    C. Decending aorta
    D. Brachiocephalic artery

50. Morphologically flattened tendon of which scalenus muscle forms suprapleural membrane?
    A. Anterior
    B. Medius
    C. Posterior
    D. Minimus

51. The phrenic nerve supplies all of the following, EXCEPT:
    A. Fibrous pericardium
    B. Central part of diaphragmatic peritoneum
    C. Pulmonary pleura
    D. Mediastinal pleura

52. Conducting tissue of the heart is modification of which one of the following?
    A. Epicardium
    B. Myocardium
    C. Endocardium
    D. Neural tissue

53. Which is the most anterior valve of the heart?
    A. Mitral
    B. Tricuspid
    C. Pulmonary
    D. Aortic

54. The diaphragmatic hernia can occur in all of the following sites, EXCEPT:
    A. Oesophageal opening
    B. Bochdalek's triangle
    C. Foramen of Morgagni
    D. Inferior vena caval opening

55. All of the following meet at the crux of the heart, EXCEPT:
    A. Posterior interventricular groove
    B. Posterior atrioventricular groove
    C. Interatrial groove
    D. Sulcus terminalis

56. All of the following are contents of the superior mediastinum, EXCEPT:
    A. Left common carotid artery
    B. Right common carotid artery
    C. Left subclavian artery
    D. Left recurrent laryngeal nerve

57. **Which is the most posterior structure in the hilum of the lung?**
    A. Bronchus   B. Pulmonary artery
    C. Superior pulmonary vein   D. Inferior pulmonary vein

58. **Which bronchopulmonary segment is prone for tuberculosis?**
    A. Posterior basal   B. Apical
    C. Anterior basal   D. Superior

59. **At which thoracic vertebral level bifurcation of pulmonary trunk takes place?**
    A. 2   B. 3
    C. 4   D. 5

60. **To which one of the following structure ligamentum arteriosum connects to the arch of the aorta?**
    A. Right pulmonary artery   B. Left pulmonary artery
    C. Left pulmonary vein   D. Superior vena cava

61. **Which nerve hooks around the arch of the aorta?**
    A. Ansa subclavia   B. Cardiac branch of left vagus
    C. Right recurrent laryngeal   D. Left recurrent laryngeal

62. **Which artery supplies cervical part of the oesophagus?**
    A. Deep cervical   B. Transverse cervical
    C. Superior thyroid   D. Inferior thyroid

63. **All of the following structures receive prolongations from fibrous pericardium, EXCEPT:**
    A. Ascending aorta   B. Pulmonary veins
    C. Superior vena cava   D. Inferior vena cava

64. **Mediastinum contains all of the following structures, EXCEPT:**
    A. Heart   B. Lungs
    C. Trachea   D. Oesophagus

65. **Whole of the conducting system is of the heart is supplied by the right coronary artery, EXCEPT:**
    A. SA node
    B. AV node
    C. Right branch of AV bundle
    D. Left branch of AV bundle

66. **The deep cardiac plexus lies in front of which one of the following?**
    A. Bifurcation of pulmonary trunk
    B. Bifurcation of trachea

C. Arch of aorta

D. Superior vena cava

67. At which one of the following sites, superficial cardiac plexus lies?

A. Behind right pulmonary artery

B. In front of bifurcation of trachea

C. Below arch of aorta

D. Behind arch of aorta

68. When the diaphragm descends during inspiration which of the following is enlarged?

A. Oesophageal hiatus

B. Aperture for inferior vena cava

C. Aortic hiatus

D. Medial lumbosacral arch

69. In severe coarctation of aorta, reversal of blood flow will be observed in which of following arteries?

A. Internal thoracic   B. Lower posterior intercostals

C. Suprascapular   D. Superior mesenteric

70. A man is stabbed in the chest with a knife which passed straight posteriorly through anterior extremity of the left fifth intercostal space. Which one of the following structures may be injured?

A. Left pleural sac   B. Pericardial sac

C. Right pleural sac   D. Superior epigastric artery

71. Which one of the following structures, lies in the posterior mediastinum?

A. Pericardial sac   B. Tracheal bifurcation

C. Superior vena caca   D. Thoracic duct

72. Which one of the following structures, may be affected by aneurysm (abnormal dilation) of the aortic arch?

A. Right bronchus   B. Left bronchus

C. Azygous vein   D. Left ventricle

73. Which nerve supplies mediastinal parietal pleura?

A. Intercostal   B. Vagus

C. Phrenic   D. Spinal accessory

74. In to which one of the following veins, thymic veins drain?

A. Superior vena cava   B. Inferior vena cava

C. Right braciochephalic   D. Left brachiocephalic

75. Which one of the following routes, a physician will choose to remove blood collected in the pericardial cavity of a patient to pass the needle into pericardial sac without entering the pleural cavity?

    A. Immediately to the right of the sternum in the sixth inter-costal space
    B. Immediately to the left of the sternum in the sixth intercostal space
    C. Left fifth intercostal space in the mid axillary line
    D. Left sixth intercostal space in the mid clavicular line

76. While ligating a patent ductus arteriosus, the surgeon must be careful not to injure which one of the following nerves, lying very close to it?

    A. Phrenic
    B. Sympathetic chain
    C. Left recurrent laryngeal nerve
    D. Right recurrent laryngeal nerve

77. Which one of the following the ductus arteriosus joins the aorta?

    A. Left pulmonary artery
    B. Pulmonary vein
    C. Right pulmonary artery
    D. Bronchial vein

78. Which one of the following veins is used in coronary bypass surgery?

    A. Cephalic
    B. Basilic
    C. Short saphenous
    D. Long saphenous

79. Which one of the following arteries is used in coronary bypass surgery?

    A. Anterior intercostal
    B. Posterior intercostsl
    C. Internal thoracic
    D. Superior phrenic

80. Which one of the following nerves is affected in thoracic inlet syndrome?

    A. C7
    B. C8
    C. T1
    D. T2

81. In labored breathing during inspiration phase all of the following muscles are active, EXCEPT:

    A. Pectoralis major
    B. Sternocleidomastoid
    C. Serratus anterior
    D. Trapezius

82. All of the following form boundaries of the thoracic inlet, EXCEPT:
    A. Manubrium sterni
    B. First rib
    C. Clavicle
    D. First thoracic vertebra

83. Which one of the following arteries is enlarged greatly in coarctation of aorta?
    A. Anterior intercostals
    B. Posterior intercostals
    C. Subclavian
    D. Internal thoracic

84. All of the following are branches of internal thoracic artery, EXCEPT:
    A. Anterior intercostals
    B. Posterior intercostals
    C. Superior epigastric
    D. Musculophrenic

85. Which one of the following nerves supplies parietal layer of central part of diaphragmatic pleura?
    A. Intercostal
    B. Vagus
    C. Phrenic
    D. Splanchnic

86. Which one of the following nerves supply parietal layer of peripheral part of diaphragmatic pleura?
    A. Intercostal
    B. Vagus
    C. Phrenic
    D. Splanchnic

87. Which one of the following nerves supplies the parietal layer of mediastinal pleura?
    A. Intercostal
    B. Vagus
    C. Phrenic
    D. Splanchnic

88. Which one of the following nerves supplies the pulmonary pleura?
    A. Intercostal
    B. Pulmonary plexus
    C. Phrenic
    D. All of the above

89. The parietal pleura is supplied by all of the following arteries, EXCEPT:
    A. Intercostal
    B. Internal thoracic
    C. Musculophrenic
    D. Bronchial

90. Which arteries supply the visceral pleura?
    A. Intercostal
    B. Internal thoracic
    C. Musculophrenic
    D. Bronchial

91. Which one of the following structures runs in the intersegmental planes of the lungs?
    A. Bronchial artey
    B. Bronchial vein
    C. Segmental arteriole
    D. Segmental venule

92. How many degrees of angle right principle bronchus makes with tracheal bifurcation?

    A. 15   B. 25

    C. 35   D. 45

93. How many degrees of angle left principle bronchus makes with tracheal bifurcation?

    A. 15   B. 25

    C. 35   D. 45

94. Superior epigastric artery passes through which one of the following parts of the diaphragm?

    A. Behind median arcuate ligament

    B. Behind medial arcuate ligament

    C. Behind lateral arcuate ligament

    D. Foramen of Morgagni

95. Sympathetic chain passes through which one of the following parts of the diaphragm?

    A. Behind median arcuate ligament

    B. Behind medial arcuate ligament

    C. Behind lateral arcuate ligament

    D. Crus of the diaphragm

96. Hemiazygous vein passes through which one of the following parts of the diaphragm?

    A. Behind median arcuate ligament

    B. Behind medial arcuate ligament

    C. Right crus of the diaphragm

    D. Left crus of the diaphragm

97. Subcostal vessels pass through which one of the following parts of the diaphragm?

    A. Behind median arcuate ligament

    B. Behind medial arcuate ligament

    C. Behind lateral arcuate ligament

    D. Crus of the diaphragm

98. Greater and lesser splanchnic nerves pass through which one of the following parts of the diaphragm?

    A. Behind median arcuate ligament

    B. Behind medial arcuate ligament

    C. Behind lateral arcuate ligament

    D. Crus of the diaphragm

99. Which one of the following structures pierces the left cupola of the diaphragm?
   A. Phrenic nerve
   B. Inferior vena cava
   C. Hemiazygous vein
   D. Sympathetic chain

100. All of the following structures pierce the diaphragm, EXCEPT:
   A. Inferior vena cava
   B. Aorta
   C. Oesophagus
   D. Greater splachnic nerves

101. All of the following structures form boundaries of the Koch's triangle, EXCEPT:
   A. Tendon of todaro
   B. Septal leaflet of tricuspid valve
   C. Orifice of coronary sinus
   D. Origin of left coronary artery

102. Which one of the following arteries supplies the atrioventricular node?
   A. Left coronary
   B. Right coronary
   C. Left circumflex
   D. Left anterior interventricular

103. Which one of the following arteries supplies the sinoatrial node?
   A. Left coronary
   B. Right coronary
   C. Left circumflex
   D. Left anterior interventricular

104. Which one of the following arteries supplies the left branch of AV bundle?
   A. Left coronary
   B. Right coronary
   C. Left circumflex
   D. Left anterior interventricular

105. Up to the level of which rib, inferior border the parietal pleura extends in the midclavicular line?
   A. 6th
   B. 8th
   C. 10th
   D. 12th

106. Up to the level of which rib, inferior border of the parietal pleura extends in the midaxillary line?
   A. 6th
   B. 8th
   C. 10th
   D. 12th

107. Up to the level of which rib, inferior border of the parietal pleura extends at the lateral border of erector spinae?
   A. 6th
   B. 8th
   C. 10th
   D. 12th

108. Up to the level of which rib, inferior border of the lung extends in the midclavicular line?
    A. 6th
    B. 8th
    C. 10th
    D. 12th

109. Up to the level of which rib, inferior border of the lung extends in the midaxillary line?
    A. 6th
    B. 8th
    C. 10th
    D. 12th

110. Up to the level of which rib, inferior border of the lung extends at the lateral border of erector spinae?
    A. 6th
    B. 8th
    C. 10th
    D. 12th

111. All of the following joints are direct articulations of a true rib, EXCEPT:
    A. Costosternal
    B. Costochondral
    C. Costotransverse
    D. Costovertebral

112. Which one of the following is related to the base of the heart?
    A. Azygous vein
    B. Tracheal bifurcation
    C. Descending aorta
    D. Central tendon of diaphragm

113. Which is the motor nerve to the trachealis muscle?
    A. Phrenic
    B. External laryngeal
    C. Internal laryngeal
    D. Recurrent laryngeal

114. Which one of the following arteries supplies the trachea?
    A. Superior thyroid
    B. Inferior thyroid
    C. Throidea ima
    D. Subclavian

115. Lymphatics from the oesophagus drain into all of the following lymph nodes, EXCEPT:
    A. Deep cervical
    B. Posterior mediastinal
    C. Pretracheal
    D. Left gastric

116. Oesophagus is drained by all of the following veins, EXCEPT:
    A. Brachiocephalic
    B. Azygous
    C. Left gastric
    D. Internal thoracic

117. Which one of the following nerves supplies upper half of the oesophagus?
    A. External laryngeal
    B. Internal laryngeal
    C. Recurrent laryngeal
    D. Oesophageal plexus

118. Which spinal nerve supplies the skin over the nipple?
     A. T3   B. T4
     C. T5   D. T6

119. All of the following are attached to the first rib, EXCEPT:
     A. Serratus anterior
     B. Serratus posterior
     C. Scalenus medius
     D. Suprapleural membrane

120. Which one of the following forms the posterior relation of the left atrium?
     A. Trachea   B. Oesophagus
     C. Pulmonary trunk   D. Azygous vein

121. All of the following valves share a common fibrous ring of the fibrous skeleton of the heart, EXCEPT:
     A. Right atrioventricular   B. Left atrioventricular
     C. Aortic   D. Pulmonary

122. How much is the distance in centimeters from incisor teeth to the pharyngoesophageal junction?
     A. 15   B. 22. 5
     C. 27.5   D. 40

123. How much is the distance in centimeters from incisor teeth to the oesophageal constriction produced by arch of aorta?
     A. 15   B. 22. 5
     C. 27.5   D. 40

124. How much is the distance in centimeters from incisor teeth to the oesophageal constriction produced by left bronchus?
     A. 15   B. 22. 5
     C. 27.5   D. 40

125. How much is the distance in centimeters from incisor teeth to the oesophageal constriction produced by oesophageal hiatus in the diaphragm?
     A. 22. 5   B. 27.5
     C. 40   D. 50

126. In which of the following parts of the mediastinum thymus is located?
     A. Superior and middle   B. Superior and anterior
     C. Anterior and middle   D. Middle

127. Which one of the following fibers are carried by the greater splanchnic nerve?
    A. Preganglionic sympathetic
    B. Preganglionic parasympathetic
    C. Postganglionic sympathetic
    D. Postganglionic parasympathetic

128. Into which one of the following veins highest intercostal vein opens?
    A. Azygous   B. Hemiazygous
    C. Accessory hemiazygous   D. Brachiocephalic

129. All of the following veins are tributaries of the accessory hemiazygous vein EXCEPT
    A. Left bronchial
    B. Left 4th posterior intercostal
    C. Left 5th posterior intercostal
    D. Left 7th posterior intercostal

130. All of the following veins are tributaries of the azygous vein, EXCEPT:
    A. Right highest intercostal   B. Right superior intercostal
    C. Oesophageal   D. Pericardial

131. Which one of the following comprises the largest portion of the sternocostal suface of the heart, seen on the posteroanterior radiograph of the chest?
    A. Left atrium   B. Left ventricle
    C. Right atrium   D. Right ventricle

132. A 60 years old patient is implanted with an artificial cardiac pacemaker. Which of the following conductive tissues of the heart had a defective function that required the pacemaker?
    A. Sinoatrial node   B. Atrioventricular node
    C. Atrioventricular bundle   D. Purkinjee fibers

133. An aneurysm of the arch of aorta may compress which of the following structures?
    A. Left phrenic nerve
    B. Left recurrent laryngeal nerve
    C. Right sympathetic chain
    D. Left greater splanchnic nerve

134. An angiograph of a patient with severe chest pain reveals thrombosis of both brachiocephalic veins. This condition would most likely cause a dilation of which of the following veins?

    A. Azygous
    B. Hemizygous
    C. Right superior intercostal
    D. Left superior intercostal

135. Blood flow to which of the following veins is most likely blocked by a tumour located just superior to the root of the right lung?

    A. Right subclavian   B. Left subclavian
    C. Arch of azygous   D. Hemiazygous

136. Occlusion by atherosclerosis in which of the following arteries would result in myocardial infarction in the area of the apex of the heart?

    A. Anterior interventricular   B. Posterior interventricular
    C. Marginal   D. Circumflex

137. A patient has cancer of apex of the lung. He has shoulder pain along with ptosis, miosis, enophthalmos and anhidrosis from half of face. Which of the following nerves is most likely compressed by the tumour?

    A. Ansa cervicalis   B. Cervical sympathetic chain
    C. Vagus   D. Phrenic

138. Cancer of the apex of the lung may affect certain vital structures which cross the neck of the first rib. This could result in:

    A. Paralysis of hemidiaphragm
    B. Hiccups
    C. Inability to close the eyelid completely
    D. Loss of sweating from half of the face

Abdomen

1. In which of the following superficial inguinal ring is present?
   A. External oblique aponeurosis
   B. Internal oblique aponeurosis
   C. Transversus abdominis aponeurosis
   D. Fascia transversalis

2. What is the average capacity of the adult stomach in milliliters?
   A. 500   B. 1000
   C. 1500   D. 2000

3. What is the length of the duodenum in centimeters?
   A. 10   B. 12
   C. 20   D. 25

4. In which of the following appendices epiploicae is present?
   A. Caecum   B. Appendix
   C. Rectum   D. None of the above

5. Which lumbar vertebra has broadest transverse process?
   A. First   B. Second
   C. Third   D. Fifth

6. Which is the most common position of the uterus?
   A. Anteverted and anteflexed
   B. Retroverted and anteflexed
   C. Retroverted and retroflexed
   D. Anteverted and retroflexed

7. All of the following structures are present in the hilum of each kidney, EXCEPT:
   A. Renal artery   B. Renal vein
   C. Urethra   D. Ureter

8. What is the mean capacity of the urinary bladder in milliliters?
   A. 100   B. 250
   C. 500   D. 1000

9. Which structure forms the left boundary of the caudate lobe of the liver?
   A. Ligamentum teres   B. Inferior vena cava
   C. Ligamentum venosum   D. Gall bladder

10. Which one of the following peritoneal folds contains the tail of the pancreas?
   A. Gastrosplenic   B. Phrenicocolic
   C. Lienorenal   D. None of the above

11. In which of the following the deep inguinal ring is present?
   A. External oblique aponeurosis
   B. Internal oblique aponeurosis
   C. Transversus abdominis aponeurosis
   D. Fascia transversalis

12. Which radiological procedure is used to study the female genital tract?
   A. Ascending pyelography   B. Hysterosalpingography
   C. Descending pyelography   D. Micturating urethrography

13. Which structure crosses the pelvic brim at the sacroiliac joint?
   A. Vas deferens   B. Ureter
   C. Obturator nerve   D. Sympathetic chain

14. At which thoracic vertebral level inferior vena cava pierces the diaphragm?
   A. 6   B. 8
   C. 10   D. 12

15. What is the length of the duct of the epididymis in meters?
   A. 1   B. 4
   C. 6   D. 7

16. The visceral surface of the spleen is related to all of the following, EXCEPT:
   A. Stomach   B. Colon
   C. Left kidney   D. Duodenum

17. Lymphatics of the testis drain into which lymph nodes?
   A. Inguinal   B. Para-aortic
   C. Subhepatic   D. Subdiaphragmatic

18. At which thoracic vertebral level aorta pierces the diaphragm?
   A. 6   B. 8
   C. 10   D. 12

19. **At which thoracic vertebral level oesophagus pierces the diaphragm?**
    A. 6   B. 8
    C. 10   D. 12

20. **Which spinal nerve supplies the region of the xiphoid process?**
    A. T4   B. T6
    C. T10   D. L1

21. **Which one of the following forms anterior relation of the left kidney?**
    A. Liver   B. Duodenum
    C. Ascending colon   D. Stomach

22. **Which of the following structures are connected by lesser omentum?**
    A. Stomach and liver   B. Stomach and spleen
    C. Stomach and pancreas   D. Spleen and kidney

23. **Into which vein the left suprarenal vein drains?**
    A. Inferior vena cava   B. Right renal
    C. Portal   D. Left renal

24. **Transpyloric plane passes through all of the following structures, EXCEPT:**
    A. Fundus of gall bladder
    B. Hila of kidneys
    C. Origin of inferior mesenteric artery
    D. Cisterna chyli

25. **Coeliac trunk arises at the level of the intervertebral disc between which vertebrae?**
    A. T11–T12   B. T12–L1
    C. L1–L 2   D. L2–L3

26. **Which one the following structure is related anteriorly to the right kidney?**
    A. Stomach   B. Spleen
    C. Liver   D. Splenic artery

27. **Which structure lies in the right free margin of the lesser omentum?**
    A. Hepatic artery   B. Portal vein
    C. Bile duct   D. All of the above

28. Which one of the following is the bare area of the liver?
   A. Cystic fossa
   B. Right lobe
   C. Left lobe
   D. Caudate process

29. All of the following muscles are present in the superficial perineal pouch, EXCEPT:
   A. Ischiocavernosus
   B. Bulbospongiosus
   C. Sphincter urethrae
   D. Superficial transverse perinei

30 Which helicine artery is primarily responsible for erection of penis?
   A. Deep artery of penis
   B. Artery to the bulb
   C. Dorsal artery of penis
   D. Deep external pudendal

31. While giving transvaginal pudendal block the needle tip should be directed towards which of the following structure?
   A. Pubic tubercle
   B. Ischial tuberosity
   C. Perineal body
   D. Ischial spine

32. Into which group of lymph nodes lymphatics of the cervix of uterus drain?
   A. External iliac
   B. Internal iliac
   C. Sacral
   D. All of the above

33. Which structure forms the left boundary of the quadrate lobe of the liver?
   A. Ligamentum teres
   B. Inferior vena cava
   C. Ligamentum venosum
   D. Gall bladder

34. The spleen is related to all of the following, EXCEPT:
   A. Liver
   B. Stomach
   C. Pancreas
   D. Left kidney

35. Which is the narrowest part of the male urethra?
   A. Prostatic
   B. Membranous
   C. Panile
   D. External urethral orifice

36. Which spinal nerve supplies skin of the inguinal region?
   A. T10
   B. T12
   C. L1
   D. L2

37. Vessels supplying the stomach pass through all of the following ligaments, EXCEPT:
   A. Gastrohepatic
   B. Gastrocolic
   C. Gastrophrenic
   D. Gastrosplenic

38. What is the approximate length of the small intestine?

A. 3 feet   B. 3 meters

C. 6 feet   D. 6 meters

39. In which of the following *Taenia coli* is present?

A. Caecum   B. Rectum

C. Appendix   D. All of the above

40. What is the dermatome in the region of the umbilicus?

A. T10   B. T12

C. L2   D. L4

41. Which defence mechanism closes the superficial inguinal ring, while contraction of the external oblique muscle?

A. Ball-valve   B. Flap-valve

C. Slit-valve   D. Shutter

42. Which defence mechanism approximates the roof and the floor of inguinal canal?

A. Ball-valve   B. Flap-valve

C. Slit-valve   D. Shutter

43. The cremaster muscle is innervated by which nerve?

A. Iliohypogastric   B. Ilioinguinal

C. Genitofemoral   D. Pudendal

44. The median umbilical fold of peritoneum is produced by which structure?

A. Urachus

B. Inferior epigastric artery

C. Obliterated umbilical vein

D. Obliterated umbilical artery

45. Which peritoneal ligament is attached to the lesser curvature of the stomach?

A. Gastro-hepatic   B. Gastro-colic

C. Gastro-phrenic   D. Gastro-splenic

46. All of the following are the boundaries of epiploic foramen, EXCEPT:

A. Portal vein   B. Inferior vena cava

C. First part of duodenum   D. Fundus of gall bladder

47. Which artery of the stomach is a direct branch of the coeliac trunk?

A. Left gastric   B. Right gastric

C. Left gastroepiploic   D. Right gastroepiploic

48. Pain from a gastric ulcer is generally referred to which region?
    A. Umbilicus
    B. Inferior angle of left scapula
    C. Epigastrium
    D. Tip of left shoulder

49. Which part of duodenum is visualized as duodenal cap in a barium meal radiograph?
    A. First
    B. Second
    C. Third
    D. Fourth

50. All of the following are normal sites of constrictions of the ureter, EXCEPT:
    A. Pelvi-ureteric junction
    B. While it crosses the sacro-iliac joint
    C. While it crosses the ischial spine
    D. Uretero-vesical junction

51. Between the twelfth rib and which one of the following structure renal angle lies?
    A. Erector spinae
    B. Psoas major
    C. Quadratus lumborum
    D. Latissimus dorsi

52. Which process of a lumbar vertebra is the costal element?
    A. Superior articular
    B. Transverse
    C. Mammillary
    D. Accessory

53. While giving perineal pudendal block the needle tip should be directed towards which of the following structure?
    A. Pubic tubercle
    B. Medial surface of ischial tubersosity
    C. Perineal body
    D. Ischial spine

54. In to which part of the diaphragm the aortic aperture lies?
    A. Central tendon
    B. Right crus
    C. Posterior to median arcuate ligament
    D. Right dome

55. Which is the most distensible part of male urethra?
    A. Prostatic
    B. Membranous
    C. Bulbar
    D. Navicular fossa

56. Which one of the following is the tough fibrous convering of the testis?
    A. Dartos
    B. Cremasteric fascia
    C. Tunica vaginalis
    D. Tunica albuginea

57. Which lobe of the prostate is devoid of glandular element?
- A. Anterior
- B. Lateral
- C. Posterior
- D. Median

58. Into which group of lymph nodes lymphatics from the glans penis drain directly?
- A. Superficial inguinal
- B. Internal iliac
- C. Deep inguinal
- D. Para-aortic

59. Which spinal segments are responsible for ejaculation?
- A. T11 to L2
- B. L4 to S4
- C. S2 to S4
- D. S4 to C0

60. The region where the labia majora meet posteriorly is called:
- A. Posterior commissure
- B. Frenulum of vestibule
- C. Frenulum of clitoris
- D. Prepuce of clitoris

61. Fascia covering which one of the following structure forms the lateral wall of the ischiorectal fossa?
- A Obturator internus
- B. Levator ani
- C. Sphincter ani externus
- D. Urogenital diaphragm

62. Which spinal segments supply the skin of the scrotum?
- A. L1 L2
- B. L4 L5
- C. S1 S2
- D. L1 S3

63. All of the following muscles are attached to the perineal body, EXCEPT:
- A. Superficial transvernus perinei
- B. Deep transversus perinei
- C. External anal sphincter
- D. Ischiocavernous

64. All of the following are branches of the superior mesenteric artery, EXCEPT:
- A. Ileocolic
- B. Right colic
- C. Middle colic
- D. Left colic

65. Which nerve is called nervus furcalis?
- A. L3
- B. L 4
- C. L5
- D. S 1

66. Which is the most common position of vermiform appendix?
- A. Retrocaecal
- B. Paracaecal
- C. Subcaecal
- D. Pelvic

67. At which vertebral level epiploic foramen is situated?
   A. T11   B. T12
   C. L1   D. L2

68. All of the following are contents of the rectus sheath, EXCEPT:
   A. Superior epigastric vein   B. Superfical epigastric artery
   C. Subcostal nerve   D. Inferior epigastric artery

69. All of the following are contents of the spermatic cord, EXCEPT:
   A. Testicular artery   B. Testicular vein
   C. Cremasteric artery   D. Artery of ductus deferens

70. All of the following are coverings of the lateral direct inguinal hernia, EXCEPT:
   A. Extraperitoneal tissue   B. Fascia transversalis
   C. Internal spermatic fascia D. External spermatic fascia

71. All of the following are coverings of the indirect inguinal hernia, EXCEPT:
   A. Extraperitoneal tissue   B. Fascia transversalis
   C. Internal spermatic fascia D. External spermatic fascia

72. Into which vein the right suprarenal vein drains?
   A. Inferior vena cava   B. Right renal
   C. Portal   D. Left renal

73. Lymphatics of the scrotum drain into which lymph nodes?
   A. Inguinal   B. Para-aortic
   C. Subhepatic   D. Subdiaphragmatic

74. The medial umbilical fold of peritoneum is produced by which structure?
   A. Urachus
   B. Inferior epigastric artery
   C. Obliterated umbilical vein
   D. Obliterated umbilical artery

75. The lateral umbilical fold of peritoneum is produced by which structure?
   A. Urachus   B. Inferior epigastric artery
   C. Obliterated umbilical vein D. Obliterated umbilical artery

76. What type of joint is sacroiliac joint?
   A. Symphysis   B. Syndesmosis
   C Primary cartilaginous   D. Plane synovial

77. Inferior pancreatico-duodenal artery is branch of which artery?
    - A. Gastroduodenal
    - B. Common hepatic
    - C. Superior mesenteric
    - D. Inferior mesenteric

78. Superior pancreatico-duodenal artery is branch of which artery?
    - A. Gastroduodenal
    - B. Common hepatic
    - C. Superior mesenteric
    - D. Inferior mesenteric

79. In which of the following four layers of peritoneum is present?
    - A. Fissure for ligamentum venosum
    - B. Fissure for ligamentum teres
    - C. Porta hepatis
    - D. Fossa for gall bladder

80. Which function is controlled by pudendal nerve?
    - A. Micturtion
    - B. Defacation
    - C. Sex
    - D. All of the above

81. Through which part of the diaphragm greater, lesser and least splanchnic nerves pass?
    - A. Behind medial arcuate ligament
    - B. Behind lateral arcuate ligament
    - C. Behind median arcuate ligament
    - D. Crus

82. Through which part of the diaphragm symphatic chains pass?
    - A. Behind medial arcuate ligament
    - B. Behind lateral arcuate ligament
    - C. Behind median arcuate ligament
    - D. Crus

83. Through which part of the diaphragm subcostal vessels and nerves pass?
    - A. Behind medial arcuate ligament
    - B. Behind lateral arcuate ligament
    - C. Behind median arcuate ligament
    - D. Crus

84. All of the following ligaments are primary supports of the uterus, EXCEPT:
    - A. Transrverse cervical
    - B. Pubocervical
    - C. Round
    - D. Broad

85. In retroceccal appendicitis extension of the hip joint causes pain because of stretching of which muscle?
    A. Obturator externus   B. Obturator internus
    C. Psoas major   D. Piriformis

86. In pelvic appendicitis pain is felt when the thigh is flexed and medially rotated because of stretching of which muscle?
    A. Obturator externus   B. Obturator internus
    C. Psoas major   D. Piriformis

87. Which structure passes through vena caval opening of the diaphragm?
    A. Thoracic duct   B. Azygous vein
    C. Greater splachnic nerve D. Right phrenic nerve

88. Flexion of the trunk or lumbar spine is brought about mainly by which muscle?
    A. External oblique abdominis
    B. Internal oblique abdominis
    C. Transversus abdominis
    D. Rectus abdominis

89. What is the combined action of internal and external oblique muscles of the same side on the trunk?
    A. Flexion   B. Extension
    C. Lateral flexion   D. Rotation

90. What is the combined action of right internal oblique and left external oblique muscles on the trunk?
    A. Extension   B. Lateral flexion
    C. Left rotation   D. Right rotation

91. All of the following are retroperitoneal, EXCEPT:
    A. Pancreas   B. Kidney
    C. Spleen   D. Abdomnal aorta

92. Which of the following arteries supply fundus of the stomach?
    A. Right gastric   B. Splenic
    C. Right gastroepiploic   D. Short gastric

93. All of the following structures are present in the deep perineal pouch in male, EXCEPT:
    A. Sphincter vesicae
    B. Sphincter urethrae
    C. Deep transversus perinei muscle
    D. Bulbourethral glands

94. A posteriorly perforating peptic ulcer will most likely produce peritonitis is which one of the following?
    - A. Greater sac
    - B. Lesser sac
    - C. Hepatorenal pouch
    - D. Retrovesical pouch

95. Into which vein inferior mesenteric vein opens?
    - A. Portal
    - B. Inferior vena cava
    - C. Splenic
    - D. Superior mesenteric vein

96. Testis is supplied by sympathetic nerves arising from which one of the following segment?
    - A. T10
    - B. T11
    - C. T12
    - D. L1

97. Which one of the following is the shortest part of the male urethra?
    - A. Prostatic
    - B. Membranous
    - C. Bulbar
    - D. Penile

98. Parietal peritoneum of the pelvic is supplied by which one of the following nerves?
    - A. Pudendal
    - B. Obturator
    - C. Femoral
    - D. Genitofemoral

99. Which ligaments maintain the angle of anteversion of the uterus?
    - A. Round and pubocervical
    - B. Transverse cervical and uterosacral
    - C. Pubocervical and transverse cervical
    - D. Round and uterosacral

100. Which nerve supplies the cremaster muscle?
    - A. Ilioinguinal
    - B. Iliohypogastric
    - C. Femoral
    - D. Genitofemoral

101. Which nerve supplies pyramidalis muscle?
    - A. T10
    - B. T11
    - C. T12
    - D. L1

102. Testicular artery is a branch of which artery?
    - A. Internal iliac
    - B. External iliac
    - C. Renal
    - D. Abdominal arota

103. Sacrospinous ligament is a degenerated part of which muscle?
    - A. Oburator internus
    - B. Coccygeus
    - C. External anal sphincter
    - D. Biceps femoris

104. **Last drop urine is a expelled by contraction of which muscle?**
     A. Ischiocavernosus
     B. Bulbospongiosus
     C. Detrusor
     D. Superficial transversus perinei

105. **What is the relation of the neck of the femoral hernia to pubic tubercle?**
     A. Above and lateral   B. Above and medial
     C. Below and lateral   D. Below and medial

106. **What is the relation of the neck of the inguinal hernia to pubic tubercle?**
     A. Above and lateral   B. Above and medial
     C. Below and lateral   D. Below and medial

107. **All of the following structures are present in the porta hepatis, EXCEPT**
     A. Hepatic artery   B. Hepatic vein
     C. Portal vein   D. Bile duct

108. **Which one of the following structures is formed by upper layer of labia minora with corresponding layer of opposite side anteriorly?**
     A. Posterior commissure   B. Frenulum of vestibule
     C. Frenulum of clitoris   D. Prepuce of clitoris

109. **Which one of the following structures is formed by lower layer of labia minora with corresponding layer of opposite side anteriorly?**
     A. Posterior commissure   B. Frenulum of vestibule
     C. Frenulum of clitoris   D. Prepuce of clitoris

110. **Which one of the following is a branch of internal iliac artery?**
     A. Median sacral   B. Ovarian
     C. Superior rectal   D. Inferior rectal

111. **Into which one of the following space vertebral venous plexuses lie?**
     A. Epidural   B. Sub dural
     D. Subarachnoid   D. None of the above

112. **Which is the important landmark for the lumbar puncture?**
     A. Iliac crests   B. Posterior superior iliac spines
     C. Sacral cornuua   D. Sacral hiatus

113. Which one of the following is the termination of dura mater?
    A. Filum terminale
    B. Conus medularis
    C. Coccygeal ligament
    D. Denticulate ligament

114. In the suprapubic incision for lower uterine caesarian section, the gynaecologist cuts all of the following, EXCEPT:
    A. Transversalis fascia
    B. Rectus abdominis
    C. Anterior wall of rectus sheath
    D. Superficial fascia

115. In the suprapubic incision for extraperitoneal approach to the urinary baldder, the surgeon cuts all of the following, EXCEPT:
    A. Skin
    B. Superficial fascia
    C. Anterior wall of rectus sheath
    D. Transversalis fascia

116. Artery of the vas deferens is a branch of which artery?
    A. Abdominal aorta
    B. Internal iliac
    C. Superior vesical
    D. Inferior epigastric

117. Cremasteric artery is a branch of which artery?
    A. Abdominal aorta
    B. Internal iliac
    C. Superior vesical
    D. Inferior epigastric

118. How many centimeters is the length of the spermatic cord?
    A. 4
    B. 7.5
    C. 25
    D. 45

119. Prostate gland is supplied by all of the following, EXCEPT:
    A. Superior vesical
    B. Inferior vesical
    C. Middle rectal
    D. Internal pudendal

120. A surgeon is looking into the peritoneal cavity through a laproscope, notices six fibrous cords radiating from the umbilicus. Which structure represents median cord running upwards?
    A. Urachus
    B. Umbilical arteries
    C. Inferior epigastric arteries
    D. Obliterated left umbilical vein

121. A surgeon is looking into the peritoneal cavity through a laparoscope, notices six fibrous cords radiating from the

umbilicus. Which structure represents median cord running downwards?

A. Urachus
B. Umbilical arteries
C. Inferior epigastric artery
D. Obliterated left umbilical vein

122. A surgeon is looking into the peritoneal cavity through a laparoscope, notices six fibrous cords radiating from the umbilicus. Which structures represent medial cords running downwards?

A. Urachus
B. Umbilical arteries
C. Inferior epigastric arteries
D. Obliterated left umbilical vein

123. A surgeon is looking into the peritoneal cavity through a laparoscope, notices six fibrous cords radiating from the umbilicus. Which structures represent lateral cords running downwards?

A. Urachus
B. Umbilical arteries
C. Inferior epigastric arteries
D. Obliterated left umbilical vein

124. Which one of the following is the characteristic of vermiform appendix?

A. Mesentery
B. *Taenia coli*
C. Appendices epiploicae
D. Scculations

125. Which one of the following is the surgeon's guide to the base of the vermiform appendix?

A. Terminal ileum
B. Mesoappendix
C. McBurney's point
D. Anterior tinea coli of caecum

126. All of the following are contents of the spermatic cord, EXCEPT:

A. Testicular vein
B. Testicular artery
C. Cremasteric artery
D. Artery of the vas deferens

127. Which one of the following receive branches from the splenic artery?

A. Lesser curvature of stomach
B. Splenic flexure
C. Fundus of stomach
D. Head of pancreas

128. Posterior wall of the inguinal canal is formed by all of the following, EXCEPT:

A. Conjoint tendon
B. Fascia transversalis
C. Parietal peritoneum
D. Lacunar ligament

129. **Which one of the following is the true support of the uterus?**
    A. Round ligament of the uterus
    B. Rectouterine fold
    C. Uterovesical fold
    D. Broad ligament

130. **What type of joint is sacroiliac joint?**
    A. Primary cartilaginous   B. Secondary cartilaginous
    C. Plane synovial   D. Syndesmosis

131. **Which one of the following is the combined action on the trunk, produced by the right internal oblique and left external oblique muscles of the abdomen?**
    A. Extension   B. Lateral flexion
    C. Right rotation   D. Left rotation

132. **Which one of the following is the combined action on the trunk, produced by the right external oblique and left internal oblique muscles of the abdomen?**
    A. Extension   B. Lateral flexion
    C. Right rotation   D. Left rotation

133. **Which one of the following is in direct contact with anterior surface of the left kidney, without an intervening fold of peritoneum?**
    A. Stomach   B. Spleen
    C. Pancreas   D. Jejunum

134. **All of the following are in direct contact with anterior surface of the right kidney, without an intervening fold of peritoneum, EXCEPT:**
    A. Duodenum   B. Jejunum
    C. Hepatic flexure   D. Right suprarenal

135. **In which of the following pelvises, the inlet is heart shaped?**
    A. Android   B. Gynaecoid
    C. Platypoid   D. Anthropoid

136. **In which of the following pelvises, the inlet is circular?**
    A. Android   B. Gynaecoid
    C. Platypoid   D. Anthropoid

137. **In which of the following pelvises, the transverse diameter of the inlet is very wide compared to anteroposterior diameter?**
    A. Android   B. Gynaecoid
    C. Platypoid   D. Anthropoid

138. In which of the following pelvises, the anteroposterior diameter of the inlet is more than the transverse to diameter?
   A. Android
   B. Gynaecoid
   C. Platypoid
   D. Anthropoid

139. Ala of the sacrum is related to all of the following structures, EXCEPT:
   A. Median sacral artery
   B. Sympathetic trunk
   C. Lumbosacral trunk
   D. Obturator nerve

140. Which movement is permitted at the sacroiliac joint?
   A. Flexion
   B. Extension
   C. Lateral rotation
   D. Anteroposterior rotation

141. Into which one of the following veins, inferior mesenteric vein opens?
   A. Inferior vena cava
   B. Portal
   C. Superior mesenteric
   D. Splenic

142. All of the following are branches of coeliac axis artery, EXCEPT:
   A. Left gastric
   B. Short gastric
   C. Common hepatic
   D. Splenic

143. Which one of the following arteries gives rise to jejunal and ileal branches for small intestine?
   A. Abdominal aorta
   B. Coeliac axis
   C. Superior mesenteric
   D. Inferior mesenteric

144. Which one of the following arteries gives rise to cystic artery?
   A. Coeliac axis
   B. Common hepatic
   C. Right hepatic
   D. Left hepatic

145. Which one of the following would be mostly affected by ligation of coeliac axis artery?
   A. Stomach
   B. Pancreas
   C. Jejunum
   D. Spleen

146. Which one of the following arteries supplies the hepatic flexure?
   A. Right hepatic
   B. Common hepatic
   C. Right colic
   D. Middle colic

147. All of the following are sites of portocaval anastomosis, EXCEPT:
    A. Lower end of oesophagus   B. Stomach
    C. Bare area of liver   D. Anal canal

148. Portal vein is formed by union of which of the following veins?
    A. Superior mesenteric and inferior mesenteric
    B. Inferior mesenteric and splenic
    C. Superior mesenteric and splenic
    D. Left gastric and splenic

149. Pain of the gallstones is referred to all of the following areas, EXCEPT:
    A. Epigastric areas
    B. Tip of right shoulder
    C. Inferior angle of right scapula
    D. Inferior angle of left scapula

150. Which one of the following is present in the fissure for ligamentum venosum?
    A. Falciform ligament   B. Ligamentum teres
    C. Greater omentum   D. Lesser omentum

151. To which one of the following veins, ligamentum teres is attached?
    A. Right hepatic   B. Left hepatic
    C. Right branch of portal D. Left branch of portal

152. Lymph from the posterior abdominal wall is drained into all of the following lymph nodes, EXCEPT:
    A. Lumbar   B. Common iliac
    C. External iliac   D. Deep inguinal

153. Which of the following nerves supply cervix of the uterus?
    A. Pelvic splanchnic   B. Pudendal
    C. Sacral   D. L5, S1

154. All of the following muscle form posterior relations of both the kidneys, EXCEPT:
    A. Psoas major   B. Quadratus lumborum
    C. Transversus abdominis D. Internal oblique

155. All of the following veins are tributaries of the left renal vein, EXCEPT
    A. Inferior phrenic   B. Left gonadal
    C. First lumbar   D. Left suprarenal

156. The lower lymphatics from the cervix of the uterus drain into all of the following lymph nodes, EXCEPT:
   A. External iliac
   B. Internal iliac
   C. Sacral
   D. Preaortic

157. The upper lymphatics from the fundus of the uterus drain into which one of the following lymph nodes?
   A. External iliac
   B. Internal iliac
   C. Sacral
   D. Preaortic

158. The middle lymphatics from the lower part of the body of the uterus drain into which one of the following lymph nodes?
   A. External iliac
   B. Internal iliac
   C. Sacral
   D. Preaortic

159. Which one of the structures, a surgeon would sever to mobilise the duodenal flexure?
   A. Falciform ligament
   B. Ligament of Treitz
   C. Hepatoduodenal ligament
   D. Greater omentun

160. In which part of the urethra Cowper's (bulbourethral) glands open?
   A. Prostatic
   B. Membranous
   C. Penile
   D. Bulbar

161. A posterior ulcer of the first part of the duodenum may penetrate the wall and erode an artery running behind it, causing severe haemorrhage. Which one of the following arteries is likely to be eroded?
   A. Hepatic
   B. Right gastric
   C. Gastroduodenal
   D. Left gastric

162. Which one of the following structures, a surgeon cuts while releasing the trapped intestine in a strangulated femoral hernia?
   A. Pectinal ligament
   B. Inguinal ligament
   C. Lacunar ligament
   D. Pectineus muscle

163. All of the following open into proststic urethra, EXCEPT:
   A. Prostatic utricle
   B. Ejaculatory ducts
   C. Cowper's (bulbourethral) glands
   D. Prostatic ducts

164. **A male patient has an aneurysm of the aorta enlarging across the left psoas major muscle involving genitofemoral nerve. This could produce:**
    A. Pain in the scrotum
    B. Inability to elevate testis
    C. Pain over femoral triangle
    D. All of these

165. **The left ureter is related to all of the following structures, EXCEPT:**
    A. Quadratus lumborum muscle
    B. Gonadal vessels
    C. Sigmoid mesocolon
    D. Internal iliac artery

166. **Which one of the following folds of peritoneum is attached to the body of the pancreas?**
    A. Lesser omentum
    B. Lienorenal ligament
    C. Gastrosplenic ligament
    D. Root of transverse mesocolon

167. **All of the following participate in the formation of the anorectal ring, EXCEPT:**
    A. Puborectalis
    B. Internal anal sphincter
    C. Deep part of external anal sphincter
    D. Superficial part of external anal sphincter

168. **At the age of about how many years, fusion of intercoccygeal joints is completed?**
    A. Twenty
    B. Thirty
    C. Forty
    D. Fifty

169. **Suprarenal glands receive blood supply from all of the following arteries, EXCEPT:**
    A. Inferior phrenic
    B. Abdominal aorta
    C. Renal
    D. Superior mesenteric

170. **What is the length of the cisterna chyli in centimeters?**
    A. 1–2
    B. 3–4
    C. 5–7
    D. 9–10

171. **All of the following veins are tributaries of the inferior vena cava, EXCEPT:**
    A. Hepatic
    B. Right gonadal
    C. First lumbar
    D. Fourth lumbar

172. Which defence mechanism closes the superficial inguinal ring, while contraction of the cremaster muscle?
    A. Ball-valve   B. Flap-valve
    C. Slit-valve   D. Shutter

173. Which defence mechanism prevents inguinal hernia, due to obliquity of the inguinal canal?
    A. Ball-valve   B. Flap-valve
    C. Slit-valve   D. Shutter

174. Appedicular artery is a branch of which one of the following arteries?
    A. Superior division of ileocolic
    B. Inferior division of ileocolic
    C. Right colic
    D. Middle colic

175. Splenic artery supplies all of the following, EXCEPT:
    A. Stomach   B. Liver
    C. Pancreas   D. Spleen

176. During which of the following, the anterior abdominal muscles contract actively?
    A. Normal inspiration B. Normal expiration
    C. Forced inspiration D. Forced expiration

177. In which one of the following parts of the liver has four layers of the peritoneum?
    A. Groove for inferior vena cava
    B. Porta hepatis
    C. Fissure for ligamentum teres
    D. Fissure for ligamentum venosum

178. Which one of the following fibers are carried by the pelvic splanchnic nerve?
    A. Preganglionic parasympathetic
    B. Postganglionic parasympathetic
    C. Preganglionic sympathetic
    D. Postganglionic sympathetic

179. Which discontinuous dermatomes meet on the scrotum?
    A. L1–S3   B. L1–S4
    C. L2–S3   D. L2–S4

180. **Which of the following pair of veins terminates in the same vein?**
     A. Right and left suprarenal   B. Right and left ovarian
     C. Right and left colic   D. Right and left hepatic

181. **A tumour is present anterior to the inferior vena cava at the level of umbilicus. Which of the following structures would most likely to be compressed by this tumour?**
     A. Cisterna chyli   B. Third part of duodenum
     C. Left renal artery   D. Right sympathetic chain

182. **Which of the following nerves contain sensory nerve fibers that convey sharp, stabbing pain in case of peritonitis?**
     A. Lower intercostal nerves   B. Vagus
     C. Greater splanchnic   D. All of the above

183. **Which of the following nerves, carries pain sensations caused by irritation of the peritoneum on the central portion of the inferior surface of the diaphragm?**
     A. Lower intercostal nerves   B. Vagus
     C. Greater splanchnic   D. Phrenic

184. **While doing appendicectomy, a surgeon should ligate which of the following arteries, to cut off the blood supply to the appendix?**
     A. Inferior mesenteric   B. Ileocolic
     C. Right colic   D. Middle colic

185. **Which of the following structures is most likely compressed by a tumour of the uncinate process of the pancreas?**
     A. Portal vein
     B. Main pancreatic duct
     C. Superior pancreaticoduodenal artery
     D. Superior mesenteric artery

186. **The internal oblique muscle of the abdomen contributes to the formation of which of the following structures?**
     A. Internal spermatic fascia   B. Conjoint tendon
     C. Deep inguinal ring   D. Inguinal ligament

187. **Which one of the following arteries runs along the superior border of the pancreas?**
     A. Gastroduodenal   B. Dorsal pancreatic
     C. Right gastric   D. Splenic

188. Cancer of the uterus can spread directly to the labia majora in lymphatics that follow which of the following structures?
  A. Suspensory ligament of the ovary
  B. Suspensory ligament of the clitoris
  C. Transverse cervical ligament
  D. Round ligament of the uterus

189. Which of the following lobes of the prostate is commonly involved in benign hypertrophy?
  A. Anterior   B. Posterior
  C. Middle   D. Lateral

190. Which of the following lobes of the prostate is commonly involved in carcinoma?
  A. Anterior   B. Posterior
  C. Middle   D. Lateral

191. As the uterine artery passes from the internal iliac artery to the uterus, it crosses superior to which of the following structures that is sometimes mistakenly ligated during hysterectomy?
  A. Ovarian artery   B. Uterine tube
  C. Ureter   D. Ovarin ligament

192. Which one of the following structures passes through the gap between the arcuate pubic ligament and transverse perineal ligament?
  A. Deep dorsal vein of the penis
  B. Perineal nerve
  C. Deep artery of penis
  D. Superficial dorsal vein

193. Injury to which of the following nervous structures may result in paralysis of the external urethral sphincter?
  A. Pelvic splanchnic nerve
  B. Pudebdal nerve
  C. Pelvic plexus
  D. Prostatic plexus

194. Extravasation of urine due to rupture of the penile urethra can spread in toall of the following structures, EXCEPT:
  A. Testis   B. Scrotum
  C. Anterior abdominal wall   D. Penis

195. All of the following structures form boundaries of the perineum, EXCEPT:

A. Pubic arcuate ligament
B. Tip of the coccyx
C. Sacrotuberous ligament
D. Sacrospinous ligament

196. Which one of the following arteries remains in the true pelvis?

A. Uterine
B. Iliolumbar
C. Obturator
D. Inferior gluteal

197. The carcinoma of the rectum is likely to metastasize via veins, into which of the following structures?

A. Kidney
B. Liver
C. Spleen
D. Duodenum

198. Which one of the following structures drains into lumbar (aortic) lymph nodes?

A. Perineum
B. Ovary
C. Lower part of vagina
D. External genitalia

199. Through which one of the following, a gynaecologist would drain pus in the rectouterine pouch?

A. Anterior fornix of vagina
B. Poterior fornix of vagina
C. Posterior wall of uterus
D. Posterior wall of rectum

200. After a radical prostatectomy operation, a 50-year-old man is unable to achieve an erection. Which of the following nerves is most likely damaged during surgery?

A. Pudendal verve
B. Dorsal nerve of penis
C. Sacral splachnic nerve
D. Pelvic splachnic nerve

201. Which one of the following nerves is responsible for ejaculation?

A. Pudendal verve
B. Dorsal nerve of penis
C. Sacral splachnic nerve
D. Pelvic splachnic nerve

202. All of the following nerves supply the scrotum, EXCEPT:

A. Ilioinguinal
B. Perineal branch of pudendal
C. Posterior scrotal
D. Genital branch of genitofemoral

203. While doing lumbar puncture, cerebrospinal fluid is withdrawn from which of the following spaces?
    A. Epidural
    B. Subdural
    C. Subarachnoid
    D. Space between spinal cord and pia mater

204. The internal vertebral venous plexus lies in which of the following spaces?
    A. Epidural   B. Subdural
    C. Subarachnoid   D. Space deep to pia mater

205. During child birth, an obstetrician gives epidural anaesthesia. The local anaesthetic agents are injected via which of the following openings?
    A. Intervertebral foramen   B. Sacral hiatus
    C. Vertebral canal   D. Dorsal sacral canal

206. Cancer of the head of the pancreas may present in an early stage by causing compression of which of the following structures?
    A. Common hepatic duct   B. Bile duct
    C. Duodenojejunal junction   D. Gastroduodenal artery

207. Which of the following organs may be spared from ischemia, in the presence of occlusive lesion of the coeliac trunk?
    A. Spleen   B. Liver
    C. Gall bladder   D. Pancreas

208. How many degrees is the lumbosacral angle, open backwards with the sacrum?
    A. 100   B. 110
    C. 120   D. 130

Head, Face and Neck

1. Paralysis of which muscle causes drooping of the upper eyelid (ptosis)?

    A. Occipitofrontalis

    B. Orbicularis oculi

    C. Levator palpebrae superioris

    D. Superior rectus

2. Combined action of which muscles causes intorsion of the eye?

    A. Superior oblique and superior rectus

    B. Superior rectus and inferior rectus

    C. Inferior rectus and inferior oblique

    D. Inferior oblique and superior oblique

3. All of the following muscles have bony attachment, EXCEPT:

    A. Procerus   B. Orbicularis oculi

    C. Risorius   D. Platysma

4. Which one of the following is a motor nerve of the scalp?

    A. Lesser occipital   B. Posterior auricular

    C. Auriculotemporal   D. Supraorbital

5. Which one of the following muscles is an abductor of the vocal cord?

    A. Posterior cricoarytenoid   B. Vocalis

    C. Lateral cricoarytenoid   D. Cricothyroid

6. Which muscle is supplied by the glossopharyngeal nerve?

    A. Stylohyoid   B. Stylopharyngeus

    C. Salpingopharyngeus   D. Palatopharyngeus

7. Which of the following venous sinus lies in the meningeal layers of the dura matter?

    A. Superior sagittal   B. Inferior sagittal

    C. Occipital   D. Cavernous

8. Which muscle protrudes the tongue?
   - A. Genioglossus
   - B. Hyoglossus
   - C. Styloglossus
   - D. Palatoglossus

9. Following muscles of the larynx are supplied by recurrent laryngeal nerve, EXCEPT:
   - A. Cricothyroid
   - B. Vocalis
   - C. Aryepiglotticus
   - D. Thyroepiglotticus

10. Where does the nasolacrimal duct drain?
   - A. Sphenoethmoidal recess
   - B. Superior meatus
   - C. Middle meatus.
   - D. Inferior meatus

11. Which muscle tenses the vocal cords?
   - A. Thyroarytenoid
   - B. Lateral cricoarytenoid
   - C. Posterior cricoarytenoid
   - D. Cricothyroid

12. Which of the following is present in the suprasternal space (space of Burns)?
   - A. Jugular venous arch
   - B. Inferior thyroid vein
   - C. External jugular vein
   - D. Supraclavicular nerve

13. All of the following pass through the superior orbital fissure, EXCEPT:
   - A. Ophthalmic artery
   - B. Ophthalmic vein
   - C. Oculomotor nerve
   - D. Trochlear nerve

14. Which of the following lies deep to the hyoglossus muscle?
   - A. Lingual nerve
   - B. Lingual artery
   - C. Submandibular gland
   - D. Submandibular ganglion

15. All of the following are intrinsic muscles of the larynx, EXCEPT:
   - A. Cricothyroid
   - B. Thyrohyoid.
   - C. Thyroepigloticus.
   - D. Thyroarytenoid.

16. All of the following muscles are supplied by hypoglossal nerve, EXCEPT:
   - A. Genioglossus
   - B. Styloglossus
   - C. Hyoglossus
   - D. Palatoglossus

17. The parotid duct opens into vestibule of the mouth at the level of which molar tooth?
   - A. Upper first
   - B. Lower first
   - C. Upper second
   - D. Lower second

18. **Which nerve supplies the superior oblique muscle of the eyeball?**
    A. Optic   B. Oculomotor
    C. Trochlear   D. Abducens

19. **Stylopharyngeus muscle receives its motor innervations from which nerve?**
    `A. Facial   B. Glossopharyngeal
    C. Vagus   D. Hypoglossal

20. **All of the following sinuses open in the middle meatus of nose, EXCEPT:**
    A. Maxillary   B. Anterior ethmoidal
    C. Middle ethmoidal   D. Posterior ethmoidal

21. **At the age of how many months anterior fontanelle closes?**
    A. 6   B. 12
    C. 18   D. 24

22. **All of the following structures pass through foramen ovale, EXCEPT:**
    A. Mandibular nerve   B. Accessory meningeal artery
    C. Lesser petrosal nerve   D. Greater petrosal nerve

23. **Which nerve is related to the neck of the mandible?**
    A. Auriculotemporal   B. Masseteric
    C. Inferior alveolar   D. Lingual

24. **The smiling expression is caused by which muscle?**
    A. Risorius   B. Mentalis
    C. Zygomaticus major   D. Buccinator

25. **Which nerve carries general sensations from anterior 2/3rd of the tongue?**
    A. Lingual   B. Chorda tympani
    C. Glossopharyngeal   D. Vagus

26. **Expression of doubt is caused by which muscle?**
    A. Frontalis   B. Risorius
    C. Platysma   D. Mentalis

27. **Expression of surprise is caused by which muscle?**
    A. Frontalis
    B. Procerus
    C. Buccinator
    D. Corrugator supercili

28. Expression of grinning is caused by which muscle?
- A. Frontalis
- B. Risorius
- C. Buccinator
- D. Mentalis

29. Which nerve lies in the substance of the parotid gland?
- A. Facial
- B. Auriculotemporal
- C. Glossopharyngeal
- D. Vagus

30. Sternocleidomastoid muscle is supplied by which nerve?
- A. Cranial accessory
- B. Spinal accessory
- C. Glossopharyngeal
- D. Vagus

31. Which one of the following nerves supplies upper incisor teeth?
- A. Anterior superior alveolar
- B. Middle superior alveolar
- C. Posterior superior alveolar
- D. Inferior alveolar

32. At which cervical vertebral level trachea begins?
- A. 4
- B. 5
- C. 6
- D. 7

33. Following are the contents of suboccipital triangle, EXCEPT:
- A. Third part of vertebral artery
- B. Dorsal ramus of C1
- C. Plexus of veins
- D. Lesser occipital nerve

34. All of the following muscles from boundary of the suboccipital triangle, EXCEPT:
- A. Rectus capitis posterior major
- B. Rectus capitis posteror minor
- C. Rectus capitis lateralis
- D. Obliqus capitis superior

35. All of the following cervical nerves supply the dura mater of the posterior cranial fossa, EXCEPT:
- A. First
- B. Second
- C. Third
- D. Fourth

36. What type of joint is incudostapedial joint?
- A. Plane
- B. Ball and socket
- C. Saddle
- D. Condylar

37. All of the following are branches of the facial nerve, EXCEPT:
- A. Temporal
- B. Mental
- C. Buccal
- D. Cervical

38. In the anterior part of cavernous sinus, the ophthalmic nerve divides into following branches, EXCEPT:
    A. Lacrimal
    B. Frontal
    C. Nasociliary
    D. Infratrochlear

39. Following are the branches of external carotid artery, EXCEPT:
    A. Superior thyroid
    B. Superficial temporal
    C. Occipital
    D. Middle meningeal

40. Lateral pterygoid muscle produces all of the following movements, EXCEPT:
    A. Depression
    B. Side to side
    C. Protraction
    D. Retraction

41 Which muscle brings about retraction of the mandible?
    A. Masseter
    B. Posterior fibres of temporalis
    C. Medial pterygoid
    D. Lateral pterygoid

42. Suprapleural membrane is represented as flattened tendon of which scalenus muscle?
    A. Anterior
    B. Medius
    C. Posterior
    D. Minimus

43 Anterior tubercle of which cervical vertebra is called carotid tubercle?
    A. Fourth
    B. Fifth
    C. Sixth
    D. Seventh

44 Membrana tectoria is a continuation of which ligament?
    A. Ligamentum flavum
    B. Apical ligament of dens
    C. Posterior longitudinal
    D. Anterior longitudinal

45. What type of joint is lateral atlanto-axial joint?
    A. Plane
    B. Pivot
    C. Ellipsoid
    D. Saddle

46 What type of joint is median atlanto-axial joint?
    A. Plane
    B. Pivot
    C. Ellipsoid
    D. Saddle

47. All of the following nerves supply the auricle, EXCEPT:
    A. Auriculotemporal
    B. Vagus
    C. Lesser occipital
    D. Third occipital

48. All of the following nerves supply the tympanic membrane, EXCEPT:
    A. Auriculotemporal
    B. Great auricular
    C. Glossopharyngeal
    D. Vagus

49. Which layer of the scalp is the dangerous area?
    A. Skin
    B. Dense connective tissue
    C. Loose areolar tissue
    D. Galea aponeurotica

50. Which paransal air sinus related to the floor of the orbit?
    A. Anterior ethmoidal
    B. Posterior ethmoidal
    C. Sphenoidal
    D. Maxillary

51. Which layer of the cervical fascia forms carotid sheath?
    A. Pretracheal
    B. Prevertebral
    C. Investing
    D. All of the above

52. Which of the following is called the danger area of the face?
    A. Forehead
    B. Upper lip
    C. Lower lip
    D. Malar region

53. Which muscle forms the oral diaphragm?
    A. Geniohyoid
    B. Genioglossus
    C. Mylohyoid
    D. Hyoglossus

54. Which one of the following muscles, depresses the mandible?
    A. Medial pterygoid
    B. Lateral pterygoid
    C. Masseter
    D. Temporalis

55. Inability to blink is due to paralysis of which nerve?
    A. Oculomotor
    B. Supratrochlear
    C. Facial
    D. Supraorbital

56. Which structure passes through foramen rotundum?
    A. Maxillary artery
    B. Mandibular nerve
    C. Maxillary nerve
    D. Lesser petrosal nerve

57. Surgical removal of which molar tooth may damage lingual nerve?
    A. Upper second
    B. Lower first
    C. Lower second
    D. Lower third

58. What type of cartilage is the articular disc of temporo-mandibular joint?
    A. Hyaline
    B. Articular
    C. White fibrous
    D. Yellow elastic

59. All of the following bones takes part in the formation of pterion, EXCEPT:
A. Lesser wing of sphenoid   B. Frontal
C. Parietal   D. Squamous temporal

60. Inferior thyroid artery is a branch of which artery?
A. Subclavian   B. Thyroidea ima
C. Thyrocervical   D. External carotid

61. Which nerve supplies the anterior belly of digastric muscle?
A. Facial   B. Nerve to mylohyoid
C. Lingual   D. Cl

62. Into which one of the following, maxillary sinus opens?
A. Superior meatus   B. Middle meatus
C. Inferior meatus   D. Sphenoethmoidal recess

63. What type of joint is temporomandibular joint?
A. Saddle   B. Condylar
C. Ball and socket   D. Ellipsoid

64. Which is the sensory nerve to the posterior 1/3rd of the tongue?
A. Chorda tympani   B. Lingual
C. Glossopharyngeal.   D. Vagus

65. Spasm of which muscle causes 'wry neck'?
A. Platysma   B. Sternocleidomastoid
C. Omohyoid   D. Trapezius

66. First cervical vertebra has all of the following, EXCEPT:
A. Lateral mass   B. Inferior articular facet
C. Superior articular facet   D. Spinous process

67. At the age of how many months mastoid fontanelle closes?
A. 3   B. 6
C. 12   D. 18

68. Glossopharyngeal nerve supplies which muscle?
A. Stylopharyngeus   B. Palatopharyngeus
C. Thyropharyngeus   D. Cricopharyngeus

69. Which nerve carries special sensations from anterior 2/3rd of the tongue?
A. Chorda tympani   B. Glossopharyngeal
C. Lingual   D. Vagus

70. **Which is the only intrinsic muscle that lies on the external surface of larynx?**
    A. Sternohyoid
    B. Cricotyroid
    C. Thyrohyoid
    D. Lateral cricoarytenoid

71. **The junction of sagittal and coronal sutures is called:**
    A. Inion
    B. Pterion
    C. Bregma
    D. Lambda

72. **Superior thyroid artery is a branch of which artery?**
    A. External carotid
    B. Internal carotid
    C. Brachiocephalic
    D. Subclavian

73. **Which nerve supplies lateral rectus muscle of the eye?**
    A. Trochlear
    B. Abducent
    C. Ophthalmic
    D. Oculomotor

74. **In which of the following frontal air sinus opens?**
    A. Sphenoethmoidal recess
    B. Superior meatus
    C. Middle meatus
    D. Inferior meatus

75. **Which nerve passes through mandibular foramen?**
    A. Mandibular
    B. Inferior alvelor
    C. Lingual
    D. Masseteric

76. **All of the following nerves pass through jugular foramen, EXCEPT:**
    A. Vestibulocochlear
    B. Glossopharyngeal
    C. Vagus
    D. Accessary

77. **Which nereve supplies the stapedius muscle?**
    A. Mandibular
    B. Facial
    C. Glossopharyngeal
    D. Vestibulocochlear

78. **Which nerve supplies tensor tympani muscle?**
    A. Greater petrosal
    B. Lesser petrosal
    C. Mandibular
    D. Facial

79. **All of the following nerves supply parotid glands, EXCEPT:**
    A. Auriculotemporal
    B. Facial
    C. Glossopharyngeal
    D. Sympathetic plexus on external carotid artery

80. **Secretion of which salivary gland would be affected if the spine of sphenoid is damaged?**
    A. Parotid
    B. Submandibular
    C. Sublingual
    D. All of the above

81. Facial nerve is functionally related to all of the following ganglia, EXCEPT:
    A. Pterygopalatine   B. Otic
    C. Geniculate   D. Submandibular

82. Which is the main venous sinus draining the cerebrospinal fluid?
    A. Cavernous   B. Superior sagittal
    C. Transverse   D. Sigmoid

83. Injury to which cranial nerve results in lateral squint of the eye?
    A. Abducent   B. Ophthalmic
    C. Oculomotor   D. Trochlear

84. Facial nerve supplies all the following glands, EXCEPT:
    A. Parotid   B. Submandibular
    C. Sublingual   D. Lacrimal

85. Injury to which cranial nerve results in medial squint of the eye?
    A. Abducent   B. Ophthalmic
    C. Oculomotor   D. Trochlear

86. Which ganglion is concerned with lacrimation?
    A. Trigeminal   B. Otic
    C. Pterygopalatine   D. Ciliary

87. Which layer of the deep cervical fascia continues as the axillary sheath?
    A. Investing   B. Prevertebral
    C. Pretracheal   D. Carotid sheath

88. Which nerve is likely to get damaged while doing lymph node biopsy in the posterior triangle of the neck?
    A. Suprascapular   B. Dorsal scapular
    C. Phrenic   D. Accessory

89. Which artery grooves the medial surface of the mastoid bone?
    A. Vertebral   B. Occipital
    C. Posterior auricular   D. Deep cervical

90. All of the following structures are pierced by parotid duct, EXCEPT:
    A. Buccopharyngeal fascia   B. Búccinator
    C. Buccal pad of fat   D. Pharyngobasilar fascia

91. Internal jugular vein is a continuation of which sinus?
   A. Superior petrosal
   B. Cavernous
   C. Sigmoid
   D. Transverse

92. All of the following nerves lie in the lateral wall of cavernous sinus, EXCEPT:
   A. Ophthalmic
   B. Oculomotor
   C. Abcucent
   D. Trochlear

93. Posterior ethmoidal sinus opens into which one of the following?
   A. Superior meatus
   B. Middle meatus
   C. Inferior meatus
   D. Sphenoethmoidal recess

94. Functionally to which nerve submadibular ganglion is related?
   A. Facial
   B. Glossopharyngeal
   C. Lingual
   D. Hypoglossal

95. Which nerve supplies the posterior belly of digastric muscle?
   A. Mandibular
   B. Facial
   C. Glossopharyngeal
   D. Accessory

96. Functionally to which nerve otic ganglion is related?
   A. Facial
   B. Glossopharyngeal
   C. Auriculotemporal
   D. Hypoglossal

97. All of the following are contents of the carotid sheath, EXCEPT:
   A. Common carotid artery
   B. Internal carotid artery
   C. External carotid artery
   D. Vagus nerve

98. All of the following lie in the parotid gland, EXCEPT:
   A. External carotid artery
   B. External jugular vein
   C. Facial nerve
   D. Lymph nodes

99. Sphenoidal sinus opens into which one of the following?
   A. Superior meatus
   B. Middle meatus
   C. Inferior meatus
   D. Sphenoethmoidal recess

100. Pharyngo-tympanic tube opens into which one of the following?
   A. Nasopharynx
   B. Superior meatus
   C. Oropharynx
   D. Sphenoethmoidal recess

101. Morphologically to which nerve submadibular ganglion is related?
   A. Facial
   B. Glossopharyngeal
   C. Lingual
   D. Hypoglossal

102. Morphologically to which nerve otic ganglion is related?
- A. Auriculotemporal
- B. facial
- C. Glossopharyngeal
- D. Hypoglossal

103. Which of the following is supplied by petrygopalatine ganglion?
- A. Lacrimal gland
- B. Glands of palate
- C. Glands of nose
- D. All of the above

104. All of the following are suprahyoid muscles, EXCEPT:
- A. Digastric
- B. Mylohyoid
- C. Stylohoid
- D. Omohyoid

105. Nucles of tractus solitarius belongs to which cranial nerve?
- A. Facial
- B. Glossopharyngeal
- C. Vagus
- D. All of the above

106. All of the following are infrahyoid muscles, EXCEPT:
- A. Thyrohyoid
- B. Sternohyoid
- C. Stylohyoid
- D. Omohyoid

107. All of the following muscles elevate the mandible, EXCEPT:
- A. Temporalis
- B. Masseter
- C. Lateral pterygoid
- D. Medial pterygoid

108. At which cervical vertebral level oesophagus begins?
- A. 4
- B. 5
- C. 6
- D. 7

109. At the age of how many months sphenoidal fontanelle closes?
- A. 3
- B. 6
- C. 12
- D. 18

110. What type of joint is present between basciocciput and basisphenoid?
- A. Symphysis
- B. Syndesmosis
- C. Synchondrosis
- D. Schindylesis

111. At the age of how many years joint between basciocciput and basisphenoid is ossified?
- A. 14 to 16
- B. 16 to 18
- C. 18 to 20
- D. 20 to 25

112. Which muscle is called the safety muscle of the tongue?
- A. Hyglossus
- B. Genioglossus
- C. Palatoglossus
- D. Stytoglossus

113. Which nerve supplies muscles of the tongue?
A. Lingual
B. Glossopharyngeal
C. Chorda tymapni
D. Hypoglossal

114. Which nerve is a direct content of the cavernous sinus?
A. Ophthalmic
B. Trochlear
C. Abducent
D. Oculomotor

115 What type of joint is atlanto-occipital joint?
A. Condylar
B. Saddle
C. Pivot
D. Ellipsoid

116. At the age of how many months posterior fontanelle ossifies?
A. 3
B. 12
C. 18
D. 24

117. How many nuclei trigeminal nerve has?
A. Three
B. Four
C. Five
D. Six

118. Portal circulation is seen in which of the following endocrine gland?
A. Pineal gland
B. Hypophysis cerebri
C. Pancreas
D. Ovary

119. Lacrimal gland is supplied by which one of the following ganglia?
A. Otic
B. Ciliary
C. Pterygopalatine
D. Submandibular

120. The suprameatal triangle overlies which of the following?
A. Mastoid antrum
B. Mastoid air cells
C. Facial nerve
D. All of the above

121 What type of muscle is temporalis?
A. Unipennate
B. Multipennate
C. Cruciate
D. Triangular

122. What type of muscle is masseter?
A. Straplike
B. Cruciate
C. Spiral
D. Fusiform

123. Which muscle is called peripheral heart?
A. Buccinator
B. Medial pterygoid
C. Lateral pterygoid
D. Trachealis

124. Which layer of the deep cervical fascia forms the false capsule of the thyroid gland?
A. Prevertebral
B. Pretracheal
C. Investing
D. Pharyngobasilar

125. What type of muscle is sternocleidomastoid?
A. Fusiform
B. Cruciate
C. Bipennate
D. Multipennate

126. All of the following muscles form the floor of posterior triangle EXCEPT
A. Semispinalis capitis
B. Levator scapulae
C. Scalenus medius
D. Longus colli

127. Which artery passes through the foramen transversorium of cervical vertebra?
A. Carotid
B. Subclavian
C. Vertebral
D. Basilar

128. Following are the muscles of mastication, EXCEPT:
A. Masseter
B. Medial pterygoid
C. Temporalis
D. Buccinator

129. What type of nerve is facial nerve?
A. Motor
B. Sensory
C. Autonomic
D. All of the above

130. In which vertebrae foramen transversorium is present?
A. Cervical
B. Thoracic
C. Lumbar
D. Sacral

131. Cervical curvature of the vertebral column appears at which months?
A. 3
B. 9
C. 12
D. 18

132. Through which one of the following, auricular branch of the vagus passes?
A. Tympanic canaliculus
B. Mastoid canaliculus
C. Jugular foramen
D. Stylomastoid foramen

133. Through which one of the following facial nerve passes?
A. Tympanic canaliculus
B. Mastoid canaliculus
C. Internal acoustic meatus
D. Zygomaticofacial foramen

134. What type of joint is incudomalleolar joint?
    A. Plane   B. Ball and socket
    C. Saddle   D. Condylar

135. Which nerve supplies palatine tonsils?
    A. Lingual   B. Facial
    C. Glossopharyngeal   D. Vagus

136. Which teeth are called eye teeth?
    A. Upper molar   B. Upper canine
    C. Upper incisior   D. Lower canine

137. Paralysis of the soft palate leads to all of the following, EXCEPT:
    A. Nasal twang in voice   B. Nasal regurgitation
    C. Deviation of uvula to the affected side
    D. Flattening of palatal arch

138. All of the following nerves supply pharyngotympanic tube, EXCEPT:
    A. Maxillary   B. Mandibular
    C. Facial   D. Glossopharyngeal

139. Irritation of which nerve may cause persistent cough?
    A. Glossopharyngeal   B. Auricular branch of vagus
    C. Cranial accessory   D. Hypoglossal

140. Stimulation of which nerve may reflexely produce increased appetite?
    A. Glossopharyngeal   B. Auricular branch of vagus
    C. Cranial accessory   D. Hypoglossal

141. At the level of which one of the following tooth, modiolus of the mouth lies?
    A. Upper first premolar   B. Upper second premolar
    C. Upper second molar   D. Lower second molar

142. Leison of cranial part of accessory nerve may cause paralysis of which one of the following muscles?
    A. Sternocleidomastoid   B. Thyrohyoid
    C. Stylopharyngeus   D. Superior constrictor

143. Which one of the following is called safety muscle of the larynx?
    A. Transverse arytenoid   B. Cricothyroid
    C. Posterior cricoarytenoid   D. Lateral cricoarytenoid

144. **Which of the following venous sinus lies in the meningeal layers of the dura mater?**
    A. Superior sagittal   B. Straight
    C. Occipital   D. Cavernous

145. **The hyoid bone lies at the level of which cervical vertebra?**
    A. Second   B. Third
    C. Fourth   D. Fifth

146. **How many degrees is the thyroid angle in females?**
    A. 70   B. 90
    C. 120   D. 140

147. **How many degrees is the thyroid angle in males?**
    A. 70   B. 90
    C. 120   D. 140

148. **How many cusps lower molar teeth have?**
    A. Two   B. Three
    C. Four   D. Five

149. **How many cusps upper molar teeth have?**
    A. Two   B. Three
    C. Four   D. Five

150. **How many roots lower molar teeth have?**
    A. One   B. Two
    C. Three   D. Four

151. **How many roots upper molar teeth have?**
    A. One   B. Two
    C. Three   D. Four

152. **All of the following cranial nerves are paired, EXCEPT:**
    A. Olfactory   B. Optic
    C. Oculomotor   D. Trigeminal

153. **Damage to which one of the following nerves would cause absence of tears?**
    A. Supratrochlear   B. Supraorbital
    C. Greater petrosal   D. Lesser petrosal

154. **Absence of tears is due to lesion of which one of the following ganglia?**
    A. Trigeminal   B. Cilliary
    C. Pterygopalatine   D. Superior cervical sympathatic

155. Cornea lacks all of the following, EXCEPT:
   A. Colour
   B. Blood supply
   C. Lymphatics
   D. Nerve supply

156. All of the following cranial nerves come out of the foramina in the occipital bone, EXCEPT:
   A. Vestibulocochlear
   B. Glossopharyngeal
   C. Vagus
   D. Accessory

157. All of the following cranial nerves come out of the foramina in the sphenoid bone, EXCEPT:
   A. Trochlear
   B. Trigeminal
   C. Abducent
   D. Facial

158. Perilymph enters the subarachnoid space via which one of the following?
   A. Cochlear aqueduct
   B. Ductus reuniens
   C. Vestibular aqueduct
   D. Utriculosaccular duct

159. Aqueous humor is produced by which one of the following?
   A. Choroid plexus
   B. Vitreous humour
   C. Ciliary processes
   D. Lens vesicle

160. Aqueous humor is drained by which one of the following?
   A. Hyloid canal
   B. Canal of Schlemm
   D. Choroid plexus
   D. Arachnoid villi

161. Into which one of the following spaces, perilymphaltic duct opens?
   A. Extradural
   B. Subdural
   C. Subarachnoid
   D. Epitympanic recess

162. Into which one of the following spaces endolymphaltic duct opens?
   A. Extradural
   B. Subdural
   C. Subarachnoid
   D. Epitympanic recess

163. All of the following are branches of the internal carotid artery, EXCEPT:
   A. Ophthalmic
   B. Anterior cerebral
   C. Middle cerebral
   D. Posterior cerebral

164. The cell bodies of the neurons responsible for pupillary dilatation are located in which one of the following ganglia?
   A. Ciliary
   B. Pterygoplatine
   B. Geniculate
   D. Superior cervical

165. Through how many openings utricle of internal ear recives three semicircular ducts?
    - A. Three
    - B. Four
    - C. Five
    - D. Six

166. Which one of the following nerves has a motor function?
    - A. Greater occipital
    - B. Lesser occipital
    - C. Great auricular
    - D. Suboccipital

167. On examining the nose, the doctor finds discharge pooling in the middle meatus. From which one of the following it may arise?
    - A. Sphenoid sinus
    - B. Mxillary sinus
    - C. Posterior ethomoid sinus
    - D. Nasolacrimal duct

168. A patient has a swelling of the right parotid gland due to cancer and he can not close his right eye. Which one of the following nerves is involved?
    - A. Maxillary
    - B. Mandibular
    - C. Ophthalmic
    - D. Facial

169. Middle meningeal artery may be involved in head injury causing hematoma. Which one of the following spaces the hematoma lies?
    - A. Extradural
    - B. Subdural
    - C. Subpial
    - D. Subarachnoid

170. Which one of the following sinuses lies below the pituitary fossa?
    - A. Cavernous
    - B. Sphenoid
    - C. Straight
    - D. Sigmoid

171. Which muscle opens the laryngeal glottis to allow breathing?
    - A. Cricothyroid
    - B. Vocalis
    - C. Posterior cricoarytenoid
    - D. Lateral cricoarytenoid

172. A swelling is just below the chin, most likely to be submental lymph nodes. Which area it drains?
    - A. Center of the upper lip
    - B. Posterior 1/3rd of the tongue
    - C. Thyroid gland
    - D. Tip of the tongue

173. A patient who has Bell's palsy, complains of food collecting between teeth and ckeeks. Paralysis of which muscle causes this?
    - A. Masseter
    - B. Orbicularis oris
    - C. Mentalis
    - D. Buccinator

174. In drinking, whlile bending over a water foumtain, nasal regurgitation is prevented by which one of the following muscles?

A. Palatoglossus
B. Tensor palati
C. Palatopharyngeus
D. Stylopharyngeus

175. Which muscle is common boundary between digastric and carotid triangles?

A. Anterior belly of digastric
B. Posterior belly of digastric
C. Omohyoid
D. Sternocleidomastoid

176. At which level common carotid artery divides?

A. Cricoid cartilage
B. Lower border of thyroid cartilage
C. Upper border of thyroid cartilage
D. Hyoid bone

177. All of the following muscles form boundary of the carotid triangle, EXCEPT:

A. Posterior belly of digastric
B. Stylohyoid
C. Superior belly of omohyoid
D. Inferior belly of omohyoid

178. All of the following structures pass between external and internal carotid arteries, EXCEPT:

A. Stylopharyngeus muscle
B. Styloglossus muscle
C. Stylohyoid muscle
D. Glossopharyngeal nerve

179. All of the following structures refract light as it passes through the eye, EXCEPT:

A. Cornea
B. Iris
C. Aqueous humour
D. Vitreous humour

180. Which one of the following nerves is most likely to be injured during removal of enlarged cervical lymph nodes?

A. Dorsal scapular
B. Supraclavicular
C. Spinal accessory
D. Lesser occipital

181. Which nerve carries preganglionic fibers to the submandibular salivary gland?

A. Chorda tympani
B. Greater petrosal
C. Lesser petrosal
D. Auriculotemporal

182. Which nerve carries preganglionic fibers to the parotid salivary gland?
A. Chorda tympani   B. Greater petrosal
C. Lesser petrosal   D. Auriculotemporal

183. Which nerve carries preganglionic fibers to glands of the palate?
A. Chorda tympani   B. Greater petrosal
C. Lesser petrosal   D. Auriculotemporal

184. Which extraocular muscle produces elevation and medial rotation of the eye?
A. Superior rectus   B. Superior oblique
C. Medial rectus   D. Inferior oblique

185. Which extraocular muscle produces depression and medial rotation of the eye?
A. Superior rectus   B. Superior oblique
C. Medial rectus   D. Inferior rectus

186. Which extraocular muscle produces depression and lateral rotation of the eye?
A. Superior rectus   B. Superior oblique
C. Medial rectus   D. Inferior oblique

187. Which extraocular muscle produces elevation and lateral rotation of the eye?
A. Superior rectus   B. Superior oblique
C. Medial rectus   D. Inferior oblique

188. All of the following structures lie posterior to the scalenus anterior muscle, EXCEPT:
A. Phrenic nerve   B. Subclavian vein
C. Subclavian artery   D. Brachial plexus

189. Which nerve runs on the scalenus anterior muscle?
A. Vagus nerve   B. Phrenic nerve
C. Anas cervicalis   D. Sympathetic trunk

190. Which nerve passes through foramen magnum?
A. Hypoglossal   B. Glossopharyngeal
C. Cranial accessory   D. Spinal accessory

191. Which structure is important in suspension of the eyeball in the orbital cavity?
A. Superior rectus   B. Levator palpebrae superioris
C. Tenon's capsule   D. Tarsal plate

192. How much is the distance in centimeters from incisor teeth to the vocal cords?

    A. 10   B. 15
    C. 20   D. 30

193. How much is the distance in centimeters from incisor teeth to the carina?

    A. 10   B. 15
    C. 20   D. 30

194. How much is the distance in centimeters from the external nares to the carina?

    A. 10   B. 15
    C. 20   D. 30

195. When one burns the tip of one's tongue by drinking hot milk, the pain impulses will be carried to neurons located in which of the following ganglia?

    A. Trigeminal   B. Submandibular
    C. Pterygopalatine   D. Geniculate

196. Which one of the following structures, drains into submental lymph nodes?

    A. Center of the upper lip
    B. Posterior 1/3rd of the tongue
    C. Thyroid gland
    D. Tip of the tongue

197. A patient complains of loss of taste sensations at the anterior 2/3rd of the tongue. Which one of the following he may have?

    A. Injury to hypoglossal nerve
    B. Injury to angle of mandible
    C. Injury to glossopharyngeal nerve
    D. Inflammation of the middle ear

198. The roof of the posterior triangle of the neck is formed by which layer of the deep cervical fascia?

    A. Investing   B. Prevertebral
    C. Pretracheal   D. Pharyngobasilar

199. The floor of the posterior triangle of the neck is formed by which layer of the deep cervical fascia?

    A. Investing   B. Prevertebral
    C. Pretracheal   D. Pharyngobasilar

200. **Anterrior division of the mandibular nerve supplies all of the following muscles, EXCEPT:**
    A. Masseter   B. Medial pterygoid
    C. Lateral pterygoid   D. Temporalis

201. **Which one of the following muscles, is supplied by the nerve to medial pterygoid?**
    A. Lateral pterygoid   B. Masseter
    C. Temporalis   D. Tensor tympani

202. **Which one of the following muscles has bilateral cortinuclear connections?**
    A. Occipitofrontalis   B. Platysma
    C. Masseter   D. Buccinator

203. **How many millimeters is the diameter of the human eye?**
    A. 8   B. 10
    C. 12   D. 24

204. **How many millimeters is the diameter of the cornea?**
    A. 8   B. 11.5
    C. 15   D. 24

205. **A patient is brought to the hospital with bleeding through the nose. Fracture of which one of the following may lead to bleeding?**
    A. Anterior cranial fossa
    B. Middle cranial fossa
    C. Basilar part of occipital bone
    D. Squamous part of occipital bone

206. **A patient is brought to the hospital with bleeding from ear. Fracture of which one of the following may lead to bleeding?**
    A. Anterior cranial fossa
    B. Middle cranial fossa
    C. Basilar part of occipital bone
    D. Squamous part of occipital bone

207. **A patient is brought to the hospital with bleeding occurring in the pharynx and regurgitating through mouth. Fracture of which one of the following may lead to bleeding?**
    A. Anterior cranial fossa
    B. Middle cranial fossa
    C. Basilar part of occipital bone
    D. Squamous part of occipital bone

208. A patient is brought to the hospital with bleeding deep in the back of the neck. Fracture of which one of the following may lead to bleeding?

A. Anterior cranial fossa

B. Middle cranial fossa

C. Basilar part of occipital bone

D. Squamous part of occipital bone

209. Which one of the following is called Toynbee's muscle?

A. Stapedius   B. Tensor tympani

C. Tensor palati   D. Levator palati

210. Which nerve supplies the skin around the angle of the jaw?

A. Auriculotemporal   B. Great auricular

C. Marginal mandibular   D. Posterior auricular

211. Which one of the following nerves supplies tip of the nose?

A. Ophthalmic   B. Maxillary

C. Mandibular   D. Facial

212. All of the following are branches of the anterrior division of the mandibular nerve, EXCEPT:

A. Masseteric

B. Deep temporal

C. Nerve to medial pterygoid

D. Nerve to lateral pterygoid

213. Paralysis of which one of the following muscles causes hypoacusis?

A. Auricularis superioris   B. Auricularis anterioris

C. Stapedius   D. Tensor tympani

214. Paralysis of which one of the following muscles causes hyperacusis?

A. Auricularis superioris   B. Auricularis anterioris

C. Stapedius   D. Tensor tympani

215. How many milimetres is the length of the nasolacrimal duct?

A. 9   B. 12

C. 18   D. 24

216. Which one of the following nerves supplies the cornea?

A. Supraorbital   B. Infraorbital

C. Nasociliary   D. Lacrimal

217. **Tympanic plexus is formed by all of the following nerves, EXCEPT:**
    A. Tympanic branch of glossopharyngeal
    B. Branch from geniculate ganglion
    C. Auricular branch of vagus
    D. Caroticotympanic

218. **How many milliliters is the capacity of the mastoid antrum?**
    A. One   B. Three
    C. Five   D. Eight

219. **How many millimeters is the diameter of the mastoid antrum?**
    A. Four   B. Six
    C. Ten   D. Fifteen

220. **All of the following are of adult size at birth, EXCEPT:**
    A. Malleus   B. Stapes
    C. Mastoid antrum   D. Mastoid process

221. **All of the following foramina are present in the greater wing of the sphenoid, EXCEPT:**
    A. Rotundum   B. Ovale
    C. Spinosum   D. Optic canal

222. **All of the following foramina are present in the cranial bones, EXCEPT:**
    A. Lacerum   B. Ovale
    C. Stylomastoid   D. Spinosum

223. **All of the following foramina are present in the cranial bones, EXCEPT:**
    A. Jugular   B. Ovale
    C. Stylomastoid   D. Spinosum

224. **Which one of the following bones is called os Japonicum?**
    A. Nasal   B. Maxilla
    C. Zygomatic   D. Frontal

225. **Which one of the following bones is called os Cheloni?**
    A. Atlas   B. Axis
    C. Zygomatic   D. Mandible

226. **Which one of the following vertebrae is called os vertebra prominence?**
    A. Atlas   B. Axis
    C. 6th cervical   D. 7th cervical

227. The basi-sphenoid joint is responsible for the growth of the skull in:

A. Height
B. Breadth
C. Length
D. All of the above

228. Asterion is a meeting point of all of the following sutures, EXCEPT:

A. Sagittal
B. Lmbdoid
C. Parietomastoid
D. Occipitomastoid

229. All of the following structures pass through foramen ovale, EXCEPT:

A. Mandibular nerve
B. Middle meningeal artery
C. Leser petrosal nerve
D. Emissary vein

230. All of the following structures pass through foramen magnum, EXCEPT:

A. Apical ligament of dens
B. Anterior spinal aretry
C. Vertebral arteries
D. Cranial roots of spinal accessory nerve

231. Through which one of the following canalicululi auricular branch of vagus passes?

A. Tympanic
B. Mastoid
C. Cochlear
D. Innominate

232. Which one of the following nerves is the cutaneous branch of posterior primary ramus of C2?

A. Great auricular
B. Greater occipital
C. Leser occipital
D. Great auricular

233. Leison of which one of the following ganglia, leads to absence of tears?

A. Ciliary
B. Trigeminal
C. Pterygopalatine
D. Superior cervical sympathetic

234. Which one of the following, would be the result of damage to the ciliary ganglion?

A. Constriction of pupil
B. Dilatation of pupil
C. Absence of tears
D. Internal squint

235. Which one of the following, produces arcuate eminence?

A. Cochlea
B. Anterior semicircular canal
C. Superior semicircular canal
D. Lateral semicircular canal

236. Which one of the following nerves hooks around the spinal accessory nerve?
A. Auriculotemporal
B. Posterior auricular
C. Great auricular
D. Lesser occipital

237. During a thyroid surgery external laryngeal nerve is damaged. This injury could result in severe impairment of which of the following?
A. Abducting the vocal cords
B. Tensing the vocal cords
C. Relaxing the vocal cords
D. Rotating the arytenoid cartilages

238. During a thyroid surgery the surgeon must ligate the superior laryngeal artery, so care must be taken to avoid injury to which of the following nerves?
A. External laryngeal
B. Internal laryngeal
C. Superior laryngeal
D. Hypoglossal

239. A man complains of numbness of nasopharynx after surgical removal of pharyngeal tonsils. A lesion of which of the following nerves would be expected?
A. Superior cervical ganglion
B. Maxillary
C. Glossopharyngeal
D. Vagus

240. During surgery of neck a surgeon notices profuse bleeding from the deep cervical artery. Which of the following arteries must be ligated immediately to stop the bleeding?
A. Transverse cervical
B. Ascending cervical
C. Thyrocervical trunk
D. Costocervical trunk

241. A man complains of dryness of nose and palate. Leison of which of the following ganglia would result in this condtion?
A. Ciliary
B. Pterygoplatine
C. Otic
D. Submandibular

242. Which dural venous sinus lies in the margin of the tentorium cerebelli and runs from the posterior end of cavernous sinus to the tansverse sinus?
A. Sphenoparietal
B. Straight
C. Superior petrosal
D. Inferior petrosal

243. Which one of the following conditions results from injury to the abducens nerve?
A. External strabismus
B. Internal strabismus
C. Ptosis of the upper eyelid
D. Loss of visual accomodation

244. Bilateral severance of which of the following nerves may result in death?

A. Trigeminal   B. Facial

C. Vagus   D. Spinal accessory

245. A 60 years old woman complains of numbness in the anterior triangle of the neck. Which of the following nerves may be damaged?

A. Supraclavicular   B. Tranverse cervical

C. Lesser occipital   D. Spinal accessory

246. The pupil of a 50 years old patient remains constricted even when the room lighting is dim. Which of the following may be injured?

A. Oculomotor nerve   B. Ophthalmic nerve

C. Superior cervical ganglion   D. Trochlear nerve

247. Afferent nerves fibers of the gag reflex are branches of which of the following nerves?

A. Trigeminal   B. Facial

C. Glossopharyngeal   D. Vagus

248. Which of the following structures contain cell bodies of the lingual nerve?

A. Geniculate and otic ganglia

B. Geniculate and trigeminal ganglia

C. Geniculate and pterygopalatine ganglia

D. Trigeminal and submandibular ganglia

249. Which of the following tonsils are called adenoids?

A. Palatine   B. Pharyngeal

C. Lingual   D. Tubal

250. Which nerve passes through foramen rotumdum?

A. Optic   B. Ophthalmic

C. Maxillary   D. Mandibular

251. A 55 years old man complains of numbness and loss of taste on the back of his tongue, progressive loss of voice and difficulty in shrugging his shoulders. His MRI shows meningioma that compresses the nerves leaving the skull. Which of the following openings these nerves leave?

A. Foramen rotundum   B. Foramen lacerum

C. Internal acoustic meatus   D. Jugular foramen

252. A 60 years old man is unable to open his mouth because of tetanus. Which of the following muscles is likely be paralysed?
    A. Masseter
    B. Buccinator
    C. Medial pterygoid
    D. Lateral pterygoid

253. A 58 years old woman is unble to open her eye because neuromuscular disease. Which of the following muscles is likely be paralysed?
    A. Orbicularis oculi
    B. Superior rectus
    C. Frontalis
    D. Levator palpebrae superioris

254. Which of the following muscles is attached to the transverse processes of the cervical vertebrae?
    A. Rhomboideus major
    B. Levator scapulae
    C. Trapezius
    D. Serrarus posterior superior

255. A crush injury to suboccipital nerve would result in paralysis of which of the following muscles?
    A. Splenius capitis
    B. Trapezius
    C. Levator scapulae
    D. Rectus capitis posterior major

256. Which of the following muscles indents the submandibular gland and divides into superficial and deep parts?
    A. Hyoglossus
    B. Styloglossus
    C. Stylohyoid
    D. Myolohyoid

257. If trigeminal nerve is damaged, which of the following muscles is most likely paralysed?
    A. Posterior belly of digastric
    B. Geniohyoid
    C. Tensor palati
    D. Levator palati

258. In which one of the following directions, nasolacrimal duct runs?
    A. Downwards, backwards, medially
    B. Downwards, backwards, laterally
    C. Downwards, forwards, medially
    D. Downwards, forwards, laterally

259. What is the length of adult pharyngotympanic tube in millimeters?
    A. 12
    B. 20
    C. 25
    D. 36

Brain

1. Posterior inferior cerebellar artery is a branch of which artery?
   A. Vertebral
   B. Basilar
   C. Posterior
   D. Internal carotid

2. Broca's speech area is located in which gyrus?
   A. Superior frontal
   B. Inferior frontal
   C. Middle forntal
   D. Superior temporal

3. Which fissure separates the anterior and middle lobes of cerebellum?
   A. Horizontal
   B. Posterolateral
   C. Transverse
   D. Primary

4. What is the averge length of the spinal corde in centimeters?
   A. 45
   B. 55
   C. 65
   D. 75

5. With which pathway the lateral geniculate body is associated?
   A. Visual
   B. Auditory
   C. Olfactory
   D. Gustatory

6. Into which one of the following dural venous sinus, cavernous sinus drains?
   A. Superior sagittal
   B. Straight
   C. Transverse
   D. Superior petrosal

7. Optic radiation is related to which part of the internal capsule?
   A. Sublentiform
   B. Retrolentiform
   C. Genu
   D. Posterior limb

8. All of the following lobes of the cerebrum have a pole, EXCEPT:
   A. Forntal
   B. Occipital
   C. Parietal
   D. Temporal

9. What type of fibers are present in the corpus callosum?
   A. Projection
   B. Commissural
   C. Short association
   D. Long association

10. **All of the following are basal nuclei of the cerebrum, EXCEPT:**
    A. Caudate
    B. Globose
    C. Putamen
    D. Amygdaloid body

11. **What type of sulcus is the post-calcarine sulcus?**
    A. Operculated
    B. Limiting
    C. Complete
    D. Axial

12. **Fibers of auditory pathway pass through which part of the internal capsule?**
    A. Anterior limb
    B. Posterior limb
    C. Retrolentiform
    D. Sublentiform

13. **Flocculonodular lobe belong to which one of the following?**
    A. Neocerebellum
    B. Paleocerebellum
    C. Archicerebellum
    D. None of the above

14. **Into which dural venous sinus superior petrosal sinus drains?**
    A. Superior sagittal
    B. Cavernous
    C. Transverse
    D. Sigmoid

15. **Which is the main venous sinus draining cerebrospinal fluid?**
    A. Cavernous
    B. Sigmoid
    C. Transverse
    D. Superior sagittal

16. **The third ventrincle is the cavity of which of the following?**
    A. Telencephalon
    B. Diencephalon
    C. Mesencephalon
    D. Rhombencephalon

17. **What type of fibers are present in the cingulate gyrus?**
    A. Projection
    B. Commissural
    C. Short association
    D. Long association

18. **What type of sulcus is the collateral sulcus of the cerebrum?**
    A. Operculated
    B. Limiting
    C. Complete
    D. Axial

19. **What type of fibers is present in the superior longitudinal bundle?**
    A. Projection.
    B. Commissural
    C. Short association
    D. Long association

20. **Into which dural venous sinus sphenoparietal sinus drains?**
    A. Superior sagittal
    B. Cavernous
    C. Transverse
    D. Sigmoid

21. The fourth ventricle is the cavity of which one of the following?
    - A. Telencephalon
    - B. Diencephalon
    - C. Mesencephalon
    - D. Rhombencephalon

22. How many pairs of spinal nerves are present in human being?
    - A. 29
    - B. 30
    - C. 31
    - D. 32

23. The lateral ventricle is the cavity of which one of the following?
    - A. Telencephalon
    - B. Diencephalon
    - C. Mesencephalon
    - D. Rhombencephalon

24. Which one of the following leminiscus is a part of auditory pathway?
    - A. Medial
    - B. Lateral
    - C. Spinal
    - D. Trigeminal

25. Which cranial nerve emerges from the dorsal aspect of the brainstem?
    - A. Oculomotor
    - B. Trochlear
    - C. Abducent
    - D. Vestibulocochlear

26. Which leminiscus originates from nuclei gracilis and cuneatus?
    - A. Spinal
    - B. Trigeminal
    - C. Medial
    - D. Lateral

27. Pineal gland is a part of which one of the following?
    - A. Telencephalon
    - B. Diencephalon
    - C. Mesencephalon
    - D. Rhombencephalon

28. In all of the following ventricles are present, EXCEPT:
    - A. Telencephalon
    - B. Diencephalon
    - C. Mesencephalon
    - D. Rhombencephalon

29. Which neurons are present in the molecular layer of the cerebrum?
    - A. Pyramidal
    - B. Stellate
    - C. Horizontal cells of cajal
    - D. Martinotti

30. Corticospinal fibres arise predominantly from which layer of cerebral cortex?
    - A. Molecular
    - B. Internal granular
    - C. Internal pyramidal
    - D. Multiform

31. Midbrain contains nuclei of all of the following cranial nerves, EXCEPT:
    - A. Oculomotor
    - B. Trochlear
    - C. Trigeminal
    - D. Abducent

32. Nucleus of tractus solitarius belongs to all of the following cranial nerves, EXCEPT:
    - A. Facial
    - B. Vestibulocochlear
    - C. Glossopharyngeal
    - D. Vagus

33. Nucleus ambigus belongs to all of the following cranial nerves, EXCEPT:
    - A. Glossopharyngeal
    - B. Vagus
    - C. Accessory
    - D. Hypoglossal

34. Substantia gelatinosa of the spinal cord continues in the medulla oblougata as which one of the following?
    - A. Gracile nucleus
    - B. Cuneate nucleus
    - C. Nucleus of spinal tract of trigeminal
    - D. Dorsal nucleus of vagus

35. In which of the following internal vertebral venous plexus is present?
    - A. Epidural space
    - B. Subdural space
    - C. Subcrachnoid space
    - D. With in the vertebral bodies

36. Through which of the following cerebrospinal fluid enters the blood stream?
    - A. Great cerebral vein
    - B. Arachnoid villi and granulations
    - C. Choroid plexus
    - D. Internal cerebral veins

37. In which sulcus middle cerebral artery lies?
    - A. Central
    - B. Lateral
    - C. Superior temporal
    - D. Precentral

38. Acoust area of the cerebrum is supplied by which artery?
    - A. Posterior cerebral
    - B. Anterior cerebral
    - C. Middle cerebral
    - D. External carotid

39. Temporal pole of the cerebrum is supplied by which artery?
    - A. Posterior cerebral
    - B. Anterior cerebral
    - C. Middle cerebral
    - D. External carotid

40. The internal capsule is supplied by central branches of all of the following arteries, EXCEPT:
   A. Middle cerebral
   B. Anterior cerebral
   C. Posterior communicating
   D. Posterior cerebral

41. Branches of which of the following artery supply the choroid plexus of fourth ventricle?
   A. Superior cerebellar
   B. Anterior inferior cerebellar
   C. Posterior inferior cerebellar
   D. Posterior cerebral

42. In which of the following olivary nucleus is present?
   A. Midbrain
   B. Upper pons
   C. Lower pons
   D. Medulla oblongata

43. In which of the following substantia nigra is present?
   A. Midbrain
   B. Upper pons
   C. Lower pons
   D. Medulla oblongata

44. In which of the following facial colliculus is present?
   A. Midbrain
   B. Upper pons
   C. Lower pons
   D. Medulla oblongata

45. In which of the following red nucleus is present?
   A. Midbrain
   B. Upper pons
   C. Lower pons
   D. Medulla oblongata

46. In which of the following dentate nucleus is present?
   A. Midbrain
   B. Lower pons
   C. Medulla oblongata
   D. Cerebellum

47. How many tooth processes are present in ligamentum denticulatum?
   A. Fifteen
   B. Twenty one
   C. Twenty five
   D. Thirty

48. Which of the following form tela choroidea?
   A. Single layer of pia
   B. Double layer of pia
   C. Double fold of pia, ependyma with vascular
   D. Single layer of pia with fringes ependyma

49. At which vertebral level subarachnoid space ends in adults?
   A. L1
   B. L2
   C. S2
   D. S3

50. Which nucleus receives impulses of taste?
    - A. Superior salivatory
    - B. Ambigus
    - C. Tractus solitarius
    - D. Dorsal nucleus of vagus

51. Which fasciculus connects the nuclei of 3rd, 4th, 6th and 11th cranial nerves?
    - A. Cuneate
    - B. Medial longitudinal
    - C. Uncinate
    - D. Lenticularis

52. Spinal nucleus of trigeminal nerve extends from main nucleus in the upper pons to which cervical spinal segment?
    - A. 1
    - B. 2
    - C. 3
    - D. 4

53. The cerebral aqueduct is the cavity of which one of the following?
    - A. Telencephalon
    - B. Diencephalon
    - C. Mesencephalon
    - D. Rhombencephalon

54. With which pathway the medial geniculate body is associated?
    - A. Auditory
    - B. Visual
    - C. Olfactory
    - D. Gustatory

55. What type of sulcus is the central sulcus of the cerebrum?
    - A. Axial
    - B. Complete
    - C. Limiting
    - D. Operculated

56. Posterior thalamic radiations pass through which part of internal capsule?
    - A. Anterior limb
    - B. Posterior limb
    - C. Retrolentiform
    - D. Sublentiform

57. Which tract is formed by ventral tegmental decussation?
    - A. Tectospinal
    - B. Rubrospinal
    - C. Olivospinal
    - D. Reticulospinal

58. Which tract is formed by dorsal tegmental decussation?
    - A. Tectospinal
    - B. Rubrospinal
    - C. Olivospinal
    - D. Reticulospinal

59. Which type of fibers are present the internal capsule?
    - A. Commisural
    - B. Projection
    - C. Short association
    - D. Long association

60. All of the following are nuclei of the cerebellum, EXCEPT:
   A. Dentate
   B. Globus pallidus
   C. Emboliformis
   D. Fastigii

61. From which one of the following ventral tegmental decussation begins?
   A. Superior colliculus
   B. Inferior colliculus
   C. Red nucleus
   D. Dentate nucleus

62. From which one of the following dorsal tegmental decusation begins?
   A. Superior colliculus
   B. Inferior colliculus
   C. Red nucleus
   D. Dentate nucleus

63. Decussation fibers of superior cerebellar peduncle has their origin in which cerebellar nucleus?
   A. Fastigii
   B. Globus
   C. Embliformis
   D. Dentate

64. Which fibers are present in the middle cerebellar peduncle?
   A. Ventral spinocerebellar.
   B. Dorsal spinocerebellar
   C. Rubrocerebellar
   D. Corticopontocerebellar

65. In which one of the following sensory nuclei of the trigeminal nerve lie?
   A. Medulla oblongata
   B. Midbrain
   C. Pons
   D. All of the above

66. What type of sulcus is the lunate sulcus?
   A. Operculated
   B. Limiting
   C. Complete
   D. Axial

67. Which of the following form choroid plexus?
   A. Single layer of pia
   B. Double layer of pia
   C. Double fold of pia, ependyma with vascular fringes
   D. Single layer of pia with ependyma

68. Inferior thalamic radiations pass through which part of the internal capsule?
   A. Anterior limb
   B. Posterior limb
   C. Retrolentiform
   D. Sublentiform

69. Corticonuclear fibers pass through which part of the internal capsule?
   A. Anterior
   B. Posterior limb
   C. Genu
   D. Retrolentiform

70. **Which nerve underlies the facial colliculus?**
    A. Trigeminal   B. Aducent
    C. Facial   D. Vestibular

71. **All of the following cranial nerves have motor, sensory and parasympathetic compounents, EXCEPT:**
    A. Seventh   B. Eighth
    C. Nineth   D. Tenth

72. **Which cranial nerve has motor and parasympathetic compounents?**
    A. Third   B. Fourth
    C. Fifth   D. Sixth

73. **Which cranial nerve has motor and sensory compounents?**
    A. Fourth   B. Fifth
    C. Sixth   D. Eleventh

74. **All of the following cranial nerves have only motor components, EXCEPT:**
    A. Third   B. Fourth
    C. Sixth   D. Twelfth

75. **All of the following cranial nerves are entirely sensory, EXCEPT:**
    A. First   B. Second
    C. Fifth   D. Eighth

76. **All of the following are nuclei of the vagus nerve, EXCEPT:**
    A. Ambigus
    B. Inferior salivatory
    C. Nucleus of tractus solitarius
    D. Dorsal nucleus of vagus

77. **Which one of the following cranial nerve decussates within the brain?**
    A. Trochlear   B. Optic
    C. Oculomotar   D. Trigeminal

78. **Anterior choroidal artery is a branch of which artery?**
    A. Anterior cerebral   B. Middle cerebral
    C. Posterior cerebral   D. Internal carotid

79. **Posterior choroidal artery is a branch of which artery?**
    A. Anterior cerebral   B. Middle cerebral
    C. Posterior cerebral   D. Internal carotid

80. All of the following arteries are branches of cerebral part of internal carotid, EXCEPT:
    A. Anterior cerebral
    B. Middle cerebral
    C. Posterior cerebral
    D. Posterior communicating

81. All of the following special sense nerve centers are located in the brain stem, EXCEPT:
    A. Olfaction
    B. Vision
    C. Taste
    D. Hearing

82. Which special sense nerve centre is located in the forebrain?
    A. Olfaction
    B. Vision
    C. Taste
    D. Hearing

83. Which one of the following cranial nerves has longest intracranial course?
    A. Optic
    B. Trochlear
    C. Trigeminal
    D. Abducent

84. Which one of the following cranial nerves has shortest intra-cranial course?
    A. Olfactory
    B. Optic
    C. Oculomotor
    D. Abducent

85. How many pairs of white rami communicantes carry preg-anglionic sympathetic fibres to the sympathetic chain?
    A. 12
    B. 14
    C. 25
    D. 31

86. Which nerve decussates in the superior medullary velum?
    A. Oculomotor
    B. Trochlear
    C. Trigeminal
    D. Abducent

87. Which is the most medially located nucleus in the interior of the cerebellum?
    A. Fastigii
    B. Globus
    C. Emboliformis
    D. Dentate

88. Which is the most laterally located nucleus in the interior of the cerebellum?
    A. Fastigii
    B. Globus
    C. Emboliformis
    D. Dentate

89. All of the following structures are seen in the interpednuclar fossa, EXCEPT:
    A. Anterior perforated substance
    B. Posterior perforated substance
    C. Tuber cinereum
    D. Mamillary bodies

90. In which one of the following axons of Purkinjee cell terminate?
    - A. Red nucleus
    - B. Dentate nucleus
    - C. Granule cells
    - D. Glomeruli

91. Which one of the following arteries supplies uncus of the cerebrum?
    - A. Anterior cerebral
    - B. Middle cerebral
    - C. Posterior cerebral
    - D. Anterior choroidal

92. At which vertebral level filum terminale ends?
    - A. Second sacral
    - B. Third sacral
    - C. Fourth sacral
    - D. Frist coccygeal

93. Tanycytes are found principally in which of the following?
    - A. Lateral ventricles
    - B. Third ventricle
    - C. Cerebral aqueduct
    - D. Fourth ventricle

94. Through which of the following cerebrospinal fluid enters the subarachnoid space?
    - A. Arachnoid villi
    - B. Choroid plexus
    - C. Interventricular formen
    - D. Median aperture

95. Grey matter of the central nervous system contains all of the following, EXCEPT:
    - A. Neuronal cell bodies
    - B. Dendrites
    - C. Neuroglia
    - D. Axons

96. White matter of the central nervous system contains all of the following, EXCEPT:
    - A. Neuronal cell bodies
    - B. Neuroglia
    - C. Nonmyelinated axons
    - D. Myelinated axons

97. How many milliliters is the total volume of the cerebrospinal fluid in the cerebral ventricles and subarachnoid space?
    - A. 100
    - B. 140
    - C. 180
    - D. 200

98. How many milliliters of cerebrospinal fluid is produced per day?
    - A. 140
    - B. 200
    - C. 500
    - D. 600

99. Which part of the ventricular system contains choroid plexus?
    - A. Frontal horn
    - B. Occipital horn
    - C. Cerebral aqueduct
    - D. Third ventricle

100. **Hippocampal formation is part of which lobe?**
   A. Frontal
   B. Parietal
   C. Insula
   D. Limbic

101. **After radial nerve injury which one of the following cells will play a major role in axonal regrowth?**
   A. Fibrous astrocytes
   B. Protoplasmic astrocytes
   C. Oligodendrocytes
   D. Schwann cells

102. **The fibers of the stria medularis thalami cross in which one of the following commissures?**
   A. Anterior
   B. Posterior
   C. Habenular
   D. Hippocamplal

103. **Which one of the following structures is related to the lateral surface of the thalamus?**
   A. Caudate nucleus
   B. Internal capsule
   C. Globus pallidus
   D. Putamen

104. **Which one of the following structures is related to the medial surface of the thalamus?**
   A. Lateral ventricle
   B. Third ventricle
   C. Internal capsule
   D. Corpus callosum

105. **Which one of the following divides the thalamus into different groups of nuclei?**
   A. Lamina cribrosa
   B. Internal medullary lamina
   C. Stria medularis thalami
   D. Lamina terminalis

106. **Thalamus acts as a relay station for all sensory pathways, EXCEPT:**
   A. Olfactory
   B. Visual
   C. Auditory
   D. Gustatory

107. **All of the following are parts of the hippocampal formation, EXCEPT:**
   A. Hippocampus
   B. Parahippocampus
   C. Dentate gyrus
   D. Cingulate gyrus

108. **All of the following are controlled by hypothalamus, EXCEPT:**
   A. Hunger and thirst
   B. Temperature
   C. Sexual activity
   D. Contraction of skeletal muscles

109. **All of the following structures divide the hypothalamus into medial and lateral zone, EXCEPT:**
    A. Column of fornix
    B. Mammilothalamic tract
    C. Fasciculus retroflexus
    D. Fasciculus lenticularis

110. **Fibers arising from the hippocampus pass through all of the following, EXCEPT:**
    A. Alveus
    B. Fimbria
    C. Fornix
    D. Stria terminalis

111. **Axons arising from which one of the following is present in the fornix?**
    A. Hippocampus
    B. Parahippocampus
    C. Amygdaloid body
    D. Anterior nucleus of thalamus

112. **Fibers of the stria terminalis terminate in all of the following, EXCEPT:**
    A. Preoptic area
    B. Anterior thalamus
    C. Habenular nucleus
    D. Septal area

113. **In which of the following terminate the stria medularlis thalami?**
    A. Habenular region
    B. Septal area
    C. Preoptic area
    D. Anterior hypothalamus

114. **How many sympathetic ganglia are present in each sympathetic trunk?**
    A. 14
    B. 18
    C. 22
    D. 31

115. **How many pairs of grey rami communicans are present in the spinal nerves?**
    A. 14
    B. 18
    C. 22
    D. 31

116. **How many pairs of white rami communicans are present in the ventral rami of the spinal nerves?**
    A. 14
    B. 18
    C. 22
    D. 31

117. **All of the following muscles are innervated by the autonomic nervous system, EXCEPT:**
    A. Visceral
    B. Cardiac
    C. Skeletal
    D. Arrector pilorum

118. What type of fibers are present in the the fornix?
    A. Association
    B. Projection
    C. Commissural
    D. All of the above

119. All of the following arteries supply medulla oblongata, EXCEPT:
    A. Anterior inferior cerebellar
    B. Posterior inferior cerebellar
    C. Vertebral
    D. Anterior spinal

120. All of the following arteries supply midbrain, EXCEPT:
    A. Superior cerebellar
    B. Anterior inferior cerebellar
    C. Posterior cerebral
    D. Basilar

121. All of the following are contents of the cerebellomedullary cistern, EXCEPT:
    A. Vertebral artery
    B. Vestibulocochlear nerve
    C. Glossopharyngeal nerve
    D. Vagus nerve

122. All of the following are contents of the cisterna pontis, EXCEPT:
    A. Basilar artery
    B. Origin of superior cerebellar artery
    C. Abducent nerve
    D. Facial nerve

123. All of the following are contents of the interpeduncular cistern, EXCEPT:
    A. Optic chiasma
    B. Oculomotor nerve
    C. Trochlear nerve
    D. Posterior communicating arteries

124. The phrenic nerve nucleus belongs to which group of anterior grey column (horn)?
    A. Medial
    B. Central
    C. Anterolateral
    D. Posterolateral

125. The spinal accessory nerve nucleus belongs to which group of anterior grey column (horn)?
    A. Medial
    B. Central
    C. Anterolateral
    D. Posterolateral

126. Which group of anterior horn cells innervates axial muscle of the body?
    A. Anterolateral
    B. Posterolateral
    C. Medial
    D. Central

127. **Which group of anterior horn cells, innervate proximal muscles of the limbs (shoulder and arm/ gluteal and thigh)?**
    A. Anterolateral   B. Posterolateral
    C. Medial   D. Post-posterolateral

128. **Which group of anterior horn cells innervates intermediate muscle of the limbs (forearm and leg)?**
    A. Anterolateral   B. Posterolateral
    C. Medial   D. Post-posterolateral

129. **Which group of anterior horn cells innervates distal muscle of the limbs (hand and foot)?**
    A. Anterolateral   B. Posterolateral
    C. Medial   D. Post-posterolateral

130. **All of the are afferent nuclei in the posterior grey column, EXCEPT:**
    A. Posterolateral nucleus   B. Substantia gelatinosa
    C. Nucleus proprius   D. Nucleus dorsalis

131. **From which of the following nuclear group preganglionic sympathetic fibers arise?**
    A. Intermediolateral   B. Intermediomedial
    C. Medial   D. Posterolateral

132. **Lamina VII of spinal cord contains all of the following nuclear groups, EXCEPT:**
    A. Nucleus dorsalis   B. Intermediolateral
    C. Intermediomedial   D. Posterolateral

133. **Which one of the following laminae of the spinal cord is concerned with exteroceptive sensations?**
    A. I to IV   B. V and VI
    C. VII   D. VIII and IX

134. **Which one of the following laminae of the spinal cord are concerned with proprioceptive sensations?**
    A. I to IV   B. V and VI
    C. VII   D. VIII and IX

135. **Which of the following laminae of the spinal cord contains motor neurons?**
    A. I to IV   B. V and VI
    C. VII   D. VIII and IX

136. Which of the following is present in the lamina X of the spinal cord?

A. Interneurons
B. Neuroglia
C. Descusating axons
D. All of the above

137. All of the following tracts are present in the anterior column of the spinal cord, EXCEPT:

A. Anterior spinothalamic
B. Anterior spinocerebellar
C. Anterior corticospinal
D. Tectospinal

138. All of the following tracts are present in the lateral column of the spinal cord, EXCEPT:

A. Posterior spinocerebellar
B. Olivospinal
C. Rubrospinal
D. Tectospinal

139. All of the following tracts are present in the posterior column of the spinal cord, EXCEPT:

A. Fascilulus gracilis
B. Fascilulus cuneatus
C. Posterior spinocerebellar tract
D. Septomarginal tract

140. All of the following spinal nerves are present in the cauda equina, EXCEPT:

A. Thoracic
B. Lumbar
C. Sacral
D. Coccygeal

141. In which part of the spinal cord white matter is maximum?

A. Cervical
B. Thoracic
C. Lumbar
D. Sacral

142. In which part of the spinal cord grey matter is much less?

A. Cervical
B. Thoracic
C. Lumbar
D. Sacral

143. The peripheral nervous system consists of all of the following, EXCEPT:

A. Spinal cord
B. Spinal nerves
C. Cranial nerves
D. Ganglia

144. Which of the following cells is unable to propagate nerve impulse?

A. Motor neuron
B. Sensory neuron
C. Interneurons
D. Neuroglia

145. Which of the following form hind brain?
A. Midbrain, pons, medulla
B. Midbrain, pons, cerebellum
C. Medulla, pons, cerebellum
D. Midbrain, pons, medulla, cerebellum

146. Which cranial nerve arises from both brain as well as spinal cord?
A. Glossopharyngeal   B. Vagus
C. Accessory   D. Hypoglossal

147. Which one of the following is the largest cranial nerve?
A. Trigeminal   B. Abducent
C. Facial   D. Vestibulocochlear

148. Which cranial nerve innervate extraocular muscles?
A. Oculomotor, trochlear, ophthalmic
B. Oculomotor, facial, ophthalmic
C. Trochlear, facial, ophthalmic
D. Oculomotor, trochlear, abducent

149. Which cranial nerve innervates the muscle, that raises the upper eyelid?
A. Oculomotor   B. Trochlear
C. Abducent   D. Facial

150. Which cranial nerves innervates the muscle, that causes closure of eyelids?
A. Oculomotor   B. Trochlear
C. Abducent   D. Facial

151. Medial longitudinal bundle connects all of the following cranial nuclei, EXCEPT:
A. Abducent   B. Facial
C. Vestibulocochlear   D. Accessory

152. Which one of the following pathways, pontine nuclei form an important part?
A. Vestibulo-cerebellar   B. Olivo-cerebellar
C. Cortico-rubral   D. Cortico-pontocerebellar

153. All of the following tracts terminate in the cerebellar cortex as mossy fibers, EXCEPT:
A. Trigeminocerebellar   B. Olivocerebellar
C. Vestibulocerebellar   D. Cuneocerebellar

154. Which one of the following tracts terminates in the cerebellar cortex as climbing fibers
- A. Trigeminocerebellar
- B. Olivocerebellar
- C. Vestibulocerebellar
- D. Cuneocerebellar

155. Axons of which of the following are efferents of cerebellum?
- A. Cerebellar nuclei
- B. Golgi cells
- C. Purkinjee cells
- D. Basket cells

156. With which one of the following cells, most of the afferent fibers to cerebellum make synaptic contact?
- A. Purkinje
- B. Golgi
- C. Basket
- D. Granule

157. All of the sensory impulses terminate in various nuclei of the thalamus, EXCEPT:
- A. Vision
- B. Smell
- C. Taste
- D. Touch

158. Epithalamus consists of all of the following, EXCEPT:
- A. Pineal gland
- B. Habenular nuclei
- C. Dorsal nucleus
- D. Posterior commossure

159. All of the following are parts of diencephalon, EXCEPT:
- A. Metathalamus
- B. Epithalamus
- C. Subthalamus
- D. Lateral thalamus

160. Fibers from which one of the following nuclei leave the cerebellum through inferior cerebellar peduncle?
- A. Fastigii
- B. Globose
- C. Emboliformis
- D. Dentate

161. Fibers from all of the following nuclei, leave the cerebellum through superior cerebellar peduncle, EXCEPT:
- A. Dentate
- B. Emboliformis
- C. Globose
- D. Fastigii

162. Which fibers enter through the middle cerebellar peduncle?
- A. Tectocerebellar
- B. Pontocerebellar
- C. Olivocerebellar
- D. Hypothalamocerebellar

163. The spinal segment C6 is contiguous with which one of the following vertebrae?
- A. C4
- B. C5
- C. C6
- D. C7

164. The spinal segment T6 is contiguous with which one of the following vertebrae?

    A. T3
    B. T4
    C. T5
    D. T6

165. The spinal segment T12 is contiguous with which one of the following vertebrae?

    A. T9
    B. T11
    C. T11
    D. T12

166. The spinal segment L1 is contiguous with which one of the following vertebrae?

    A. T10
    B. T11
    C. T12
    D. L1

167. The spinal segment L5 is contiguous with which one of the following vertebrae?

    A. T12
    B. L1
    C. L3
    D. L5

168. Sacral and coccygeal spinal segments are contiguous with which one of the following vertebrae?

    A. L1
    B. L3
    C. L5
    D. S1

169. Which one of the following spinal nerves does not supply any area of the skin?

    A. C1
    B. L5
    C. S1
    D. S5

170. Arteria radicularis magna (artery of Adamkiewicz) usually arises from which one of the following arteries?

    A. 5th intercostal
    B. 11th intercostal
    C. 5th lumbar
    D. Sacral

171. Which one of the following is the inferior contination of the pia mater of spinal cord?

    A. Conus medullaris
    B. Cauda equina
    C. Ganglion impar
    D. Filum terminale

172. Which one of the following forms bulb of the posterior horn of the lateral ventricle?

    A. Optic raditations
    B. Superior longitudinal fasciculus
    C. Forceps minor
    D. Forceps major

173. Extension of which one of the following cells forms the perivascular foot of the blood–brain barrier?
    A. Microglia
    B. Ependymal cells
    C. Oligodendrocytes
    D. Astrocytes

174. In which one of the following parts of the spinal cord, lower motor neurons are located?
    A. Anterior grey column
    B. Posterior grey column
    C. Lateral grey column
    D. Grey commissure

175. The somatic efferent cells of ventral grey column of the spinal cord are known as:
    A. Ganglion cells
    B. Gamma motor neurons
    C. Alpha motor neurons
    D. Renshaw cells

176. From which one of the following fibers of posterior spino-cerebellar tract arise?
    A. Nucleus proprius
    B. Nucleus dorsalis
    C. Substantia gelatinosa
    D. Intermediomedial nucleus

177. From which one of the following fibers of ventral and lateral spinothalamic tracts arise?
    A. Nucleus proprius
    B. Nucleus dorsalis
    C. Substantia gelatinosa
    D. Intermediomedial nucleus

178. From which one of the following fibers of medial reticulo-spinal tract begin?
    A. Diencephalon
    B. Midbrain
    C. Pons
    D. Medulla oblongata

179. From which one of the following fibers of lateral reticulo-spinal tract begin?
    A. Diencephalon
    B. Midbrain
    C. Pons
    D. Medulla oblongata

180. In which one of the following descending autononic fibers originate?
    A. Cerebral cortex area 4
    B. Mid brain
    C. Thalamus
    D. Hypothalamus

181. In which one of the following, tectospinal fibers originate?
    A. Cerebral cortex area 4
    B. Thalamus
    C. Superior colliculus
    D. Inferior colliculus

182. Cerebral peduncle is made up of all of the following parts, EXCEPT:
     A. Crus cerebri
     B. Substantia nigra
     C. Tegmentum
     D. Tectum

183. Which one of the following nuclei of the hypothalamus synthesizes antidiuretic hormone?
     A. Preoptic
     B. Supraoptic
     C. Suprachiasmatic
     D. Paraventricular

184. Which one of the following nuclei of the hypothalamus synthesizes oxytocin hormone?
     A. Preoptic
     B. Supraoptic
     C. Suprachiasmatic
     D. Paraventricular

185. All of the following sulci are present on the medial surface of the cerebrum, EXCEPT:
     A. Cingulate
     B. Callossal
     C. Parieto-occipital
     D. Interparietal

186. Which of the following olfactory stria carry most of the axons of the olfactory tract?
     A. Medial olfactory stria
     B. Lateral olfactory stria
     C. Intermediate olfactory stria
     D. All of the above

187. All of the following are involved in the auditory pathway, EXCEPT:
     A. Cochlear nuclei
     B. Medial geniculate body
     C. Inferior olivary nucleus
     D. Inferior colliculus

188. All of the following structures are seen in the floor of the fourth ventricle, EXCEPT:
     A. Median sulcus
     B. Sulcus limitans
     C. Stria medularis
     D. Stria terminalis

189. All of the following veins are tributaries of the internal cerebral vein, EXCEPT:
     A. Septal
     B. Great cerebral
     C. Choroidal
     D. Thalamostriate

190. The medulla oblongata is supplied by all of the following arteries, EXCEPT:
     A. Anterior spinal
     B. Posterior spinal
     C. Anterior inferior cerebellar
     D. Posterior inferior cerebellar

191. The pons is supplied by all of the following arteries, EXCEPT:
    A. Basilar
    B. Superior cerebellar
    C. Anterior inferior cerebellar
    D. Posterior inferior cerebellar

192. The midbrain is supplied by all of the following arteries, EXCEPT:
    A. Basilar
    B. Superior cerebellar
    C. Anterior inferior cerebellar
    D. Posterior cerebral

193. Which of the following motor and sensory areas of the cerebral cortex are supplied by cortical branches of the anterior cerebral artery?
    A. Face
    B. Neck
    C. Hand
    D. Perineum

194. What type of sulcus is precalcarine sulcus?
    A. Complete
    B. Axial
    C. Operculated
    D. Secondary

195. What type of sulcus is lateral sulcus?
    A. Complete
    B. Axial
    C. Operculated
    D. Secondary

196. What type of sulcus is parieto-occipital sulcus?
    A. Complete
    B. Axial
    C. Operculated
    D. Secondary

197. On which one of the following thalamic nuclei, spinothalamic tracts terminate?
    A. Ventral posteromedial
    B. Ventral posterolateral
    C. Ventral lateral
    D. Pulvinar

198. Which one of the following arteries supplies the temporal pole of the cerebrum?
    A. Anterior cerebral
    B. Middle cerebral
    C. Posterior cerebral
    D. Anterior communicting

199. Which one of the following nerves is the branch of the geniculate ganglion?
    A. Greater petrosal
    B. Lesser petrosal
    C. Chorda tympani
    D. Nerve to stapedius

200. Which one of the following arteries lies in the pontine cistern?
    A. Superior cerebellar
    B. Anterior inferior cerebellar
    C. Basilar
    D. Posterior cerebral

Embryology

1. Which weeks of intrauterine life are considered as critical period of human development?
   - A. 1 to 4
   - B. 2 to 6
   - C. 3 to 8
   - D. 6 to 12

2. Which structure is derived from neural crest?
   - A. Cerebrum
   - B. Spinal cord
   - C. Microglia
   - D. Melanocytes

3. Maternal part of placenta develops from which one of the following?
   - A. Decidua capsularis
   - B. Decidua basalis
   - C. Decidua parietalis
   - D. Chorion frondosum

4. Which mesoderm forms somites?
   - A. Paraxial
   - B. Intermediate
   - C. Lateral plate
   - D. Extraembryonic

5. Which is the nerve of third pharyngeal arch?
   - A. Glossopharyngeal
   - B. Superior laryngeal
   - C. Recurrent laryngeal
   - D. Pharyngeal branch of vagus

6. During spermatogenesis reduction division occurs in which of the following cell?
   - A. Spermatogonium
   - B. Primary spermatocyte
   - C. Secondary spermatocyte
   - D. Spermatid

7. Up to end of which intrauterine week is called embryonic period?
   - A. 4th
   - B. 8th
   - C. 12th
   - D. 16th

8. Spermatozoa undergo a period maturation for about 7 hr after ejaculation is called:
   - A. Compaction
   - B. Cleavage
   - C. Capacitation
   - D. Spermeation

9. Which pharyngeal pouch gives rise to palatine tonsil?
   A. First   B. Second
   C. Third   D. Fourth

10. What is the derivative of mesonephric duct in the females?
    A. Round ligament of ovary   B. Fallopian tube
    C. Upper part of vagina   D. Ureter

11 Acrosomal cap of the sperm is formed by which organelle?
   A. Mitochondria   B. Endoplasmic reticulum
   C. Nucleus   D. Golgi apparatus

12. Nucleus pulposus is a remnant of which one of the following structures?
    A. Primitive streak   B. Neural tube
    C. Notochord   D. Neural crest

13. In which week of intrauterine life primitive uteroplacental circulation is established?
    A. 1st   B. 2nd
    C. 3rd   D. 4th

14. Foetal part of placenta is developed from which one of the following structures?
    A. Chorion laevae   B. Decidua basalis
    C. Chorion frondosum   D. Decidual parietalis

15. From which septum fossa ovalis develops?
    A. Primum   B. Secundum
    C. Intermedium   D. Spurium

16. All of the following are derivatives of the foregut, EXCEPT:
    A. Liver   B. Stomach
    C. 3rd part of duodenum   D. Lung

17. From which germ layer enamel of the tooth develops?
    A. Surface ectoderm   B. Neuro ectoderm
    C. Mesoderm   D. Endoderm

18. Which is the nerve of the first pharyngeal arch?
    A. Maxillary   B. Facial
    C. Mandibular   D. Glossopharyngeal

19. What is the skeletal element of second branchial arch?
    A. Malleus   B. Stapes
    C. Incus   D. Mandible

20. During oogenesis reduction division occurs is which one of the following cells?
    A. Oogonium
    B. Primary oocyte
    C. Secondary oocyte
    D. Ovum

21. By which day of intrauterine life bilaminar embryonic disc is formed?
    A. 6
    B. 8
    C. 10
    D. 12

22. In how many days spermatogenesis is completed?
    A. 30 to 34
    B. 60 to 64
    C. 90 to 94
    D. 120 to 124

23. What is the normal site of fertilization?
    A. Infundibulm of uterine tube
    B. Vagina
    C. Ampulla of uterine tube
    D. Uterus

24. All of the following are derivatives of mid gut, EXCEPT:
    A. Caecum
    B. Appendix
    C. Descending colon
    D. Jejunum

25. From which of the following placenta develops?
    A. Chorion laevae and decidua basalis
    B. Chorion frondosum and decidua parietalis
    C. Chorion frondosum and decidua basalis
    D. Chorion laevae and decidua capsularis

26. From which structure secretary part of the kidney develops?
    A. Pronephros
    B. Mesonephros
    C. Metanephros
    D. All of the above

27. All of the following are derivatives of hind gut, EXCEPT:
    A. Caecum
    B. Descending colon
    C. Rectum
    D. Sigmoid colon

28. Which is the nerve of the second pharyngeal arch?
    A. Maxillary
    B. Mandibular.
    C. Facial
    D. Glossopharyngeal

29. Which is the nerve of the fourth pharyngeal arch?
    A. Glossopharyngeal
    B. Superior laryngeal
    C. Recurrent laryngeal
    D. Facial

30. The thymus gland develops from which pharyngeal pouch?
    A. First
    B. Second
    C. Third
    D. Fourth

31. All of the following are derivatives of first pharyngeal arch, EXCEPT:
    A. Malleus
    B. Incus
    C. Stapes
    D. Spine of sphenoid

32. Hyoid bone develops from which pharyngeal arches?
    A. First and second
    B. Second and third
    C. Third and fourth
    D. Fourth and sixth

33. Cartilaginous components of which pharyngeal arches give rise to laryngeal cartilages?
    A. First and second
    B. Second and third
    C. Third and fourth
    D. Fourth and sixth

34. Stylopharyngeus muscle develops from which pharyngeal arch?
    A. First
    B. Second
    C. Third
    D. Fourth

35. From which duct uterus develops?
    A. Pronephric
    B. Mesonephric
    C. Metanephric
    D. Paramesonephric

36. Which ligament is a derivative of the first pharyngeal arch cartilage?
    A. Stylomandibular
    B. Stylohyoid
    C. Sphenomandibular
    D. Pterygomandibular

37. Which ligament is a derivative of the second pharyngeal arch cartilage?
    A. Stylomandibular
    B. Stylohyoid
    C. Sphenomandibular
    C. Pterygomandibular

38. Sphenomandibular ligament is a derivative of which pharyngeal arch cartilage?
    A. First
    B. Second
    C. Third
    D. Fourth

39. Stylohyoid ligament is a derivative of which pharyngeal arch cartilage?
    A. First
    B. Second
    C. Third
    D. Fourth

40. From which germ layer sphincter pupillae muscle develops?
- A. Surface ectoderm
- B. Neuroectoderm
- C. Somatopleuric mesoderm
- D. Splanchnopleuric mesoderm

41. From which germ layer epidermis of the skin develops?
- A. Surface ectoderm
- B. Neuroectoderm
- C. Mesoderm
- D. Endoderm

42. From which germ layer dermis of the skin develops?
- A. Surface ectoderm
- B. Neuroectoderm
- C. Mesoderm
- D. Endoderm

43. From which germ layer lens of the eye develops?
- A. Surface ectoderm
- B. Neuroectoderm
- C. Mesoderm
- D. Endoderm

44. From which brain vesicle medulla oblongata develops?
- A. Mesencephalon
- B. Metencephalon
- C. Myelencephalon
- D. Diencephalon

45. From which brain vesicle pons develops?
- A. Mesencephalon
- B. Metencephalon
- C. Myelencephalon
- D. Diencephalon

46. From which brain vesicle cerebellum develops?
- A. Diencephalon
- B. Mesencephalon
- C. Metencephalon
- D. Myelencephalon

47. From which brain vesicle cerebrum develops?
- A. Telencephalon
- B. Diencephalon
- C. Mesencephalon
- D. Rhombencephalon

48. From which brain vesicle midbrain develops?
- A. Diencephalon
- B. Mesencephalon
- C. Metencephalon
- D. Myelencephalon

49. All of the following are seen in Fallot's tetralogy, EXCEPT:
- A . Pulmonary stenosis
- B. Overriding of aorta
- C. Ventricular septal defect
- D. Left ventricular hypertrophy

50. All of the following are derivatives of midgut, EXCEPT:
- A. First part duodenum
- B. Jejunum
- C. Ileum
- D. Caecum

51. Primitive streak develops in which week of intrauterine life?
    A. 2nd
    B. 3rd
    C. 4th
    D. 5th

52. Notochord develops in which week of intrauterine life?
    A. 2nd
    B. 3rd
    C. 4th
    D. 5th

53. Yolk sac develops in which week of intrauterine life?
    A. 2nd
    B. 3rd
    C. 4th
    D. 5th

54. Amnion develops in which week of intrauterine life?
    A. 2nd
    B. 3rd
    C. 4th
    D. 5th

55. All of the following are derivatives of neural crest cells, EXCEPT:
    A. Dura mater
    B. Arachnoid mater
    C. Pia mater
    D. Melanocyte

56. Dentine of tooth develops from which germ layer?
    A. Surface ectoderm
    B. Neuroectoderm
    C. Mesoderm
    D. Endoderm

57. From which brain vesicle thalamus develops?
    A. Telencephalon
    B. Diencephalon
    C. Mesencephalon
    D. Rhombencephalon

58. Cerebral aqueduct is a cavity of which brain vesicle?
    A. Telencephalon
    B. Diencephalon
    C. Mesencephalon
    D. Rhombencephalon

59. Lateral ventricle is a cavity of which brain vesicle?
    A. Telencephalon
    B. Diencephalon
    C. Mesencephalon
    D. Rhombencephalon

60. Fourth ventricle is a cavity of which brain vesicle?
    A. Telencephalon
    B. Diencephalon
    C. Mesencephalon
    D. Rhombencephalon

61. Third ventricle is a cavity of which brain vesicle?
    A. Telencephalon
    B. Diencephalon
    C. Mesencephalon
    D. Rhombencephalon

62. From which germ layer root of the tooth develops?

A. Surface ectoderm
B. Neuroectoderm
C. Mesoderm
D. Endoderm

63. From which germ layer cementum of the tooth develops?

A. Surface ectoderm
B. Neuroectoderm
C. Mesoderm
D. Endoderm

64. From which germ layer mammary gland develops?

A. Surface ectoderm
B. Neuroectoderm
C. Mesoderm
D. Endoderm

65. From which germ layer sebaceous gland develops?

A. Surface ectoderm
B. Neuroectoderm
C. Mesoderm
D. Endoderm

66. What is the derivative of the ultimobranchial body?

A. Parafollicular cells of thyroid
B. Thymus
C. Parathyroid
D. Follicular cells of thyroid

67. Primordial germ cells are formed on which structure?

A. Amnion
B. Yolk sac
C. Gonads
D. Chorion

68. During development of heart the left venous valve and septum spurium fuse with which septum?

A. Spiral
B. Interventricular
C. Interatrial
D. Atrioventricular

69. Occipitofrontalis muscle develops from which pharyngeal arch?

A. First
B. Second
C. Third
D. Fourth

70. Styloid process develops from which pharyngeal arch?

A. First
B. Second
C. Third
D. Fourth

71 Anterior belly of digastric muscle develops from which pharyngeal arch?

A. First
B. Second
C. Third
D. Fourth

72. **Posterior belly of digastric muscle develops from which pharyngeal arch?**
    - A. First
    - B. Second
    - C. Third
    - D. Fourth

73. **Thyroid cartilage develops from which pharyngeal arch?**
    - A. First
    - B. Second
    - C. Third
    - D. Fourth and sixth

74. **Superior parathyroid glands develop from which pharyngeal pouch?**
    - A. Ventral part of third
    - B. Dorsal part of third
    - C. Ventral part of fourth
    - D. Dorsal part of fourth

75. **Inferior parathyroid glands develops from which pharyngeal pouch?**
    - A. Ventral part of third
    - B. Dorsal part of third
    - C. Ventral part of fourth
    - D. Dorsal part of fourth

76. **Which is the pretrematic nerve of the first pharyngeal arch?**
    - A. Lingual
    - B. Chorda tympani
    - C. Maxillary
    - D. Glossopharyngeal

77. **Middle ear cavity develops from which pharyngeal pouch?**
    - A. First
    - B. Second
    - C. Third
    - D. Fourth

78. **Pharyngotympanic tube develops from which pharyngeal pouch?**
    - A. First
    - B. Second
    - C. Third
    - D. Fourth

79. **Smooth part of right atrium is formed by which of the following?**
    - A. Right half of the primitive atrium
    - B. Right horn of sinus venosus
    - C. Right half of the atrioventricular septum
    - D. Interatrial septum

80. **From which germ layer parotid gland develops?**
    - A. Neuroectoderm
    - B. Surface ectoderm
    - C. Mesoderm
    - D. Endoderm

81. **From which germ layer submandibular gland develops?**
    - A. Neuroectoderm
    - B. Surface ectoderm
    - C. Mesoderm
    - D. Endoderm

82. Which congenital anomaly is associated with oligohydram-
    nios?
    A. Renal agenesis   B. Tracheoesophageal fistula
    C. Anencephaly   D. Imperforate anus

83. Which congenital anomaly is associated with polyhydram-
    nios?
    A. Renal agenesis   B. Oesophageal atresia
    C. Fallot's tetralogy   C. Malrotation of gut

84. Which structure is derived form the left horn of the sinus
    venosus?
    A. Oblique vein of the left atrium
    B. Smooth part of the left atrium
    C. Rough part of left atrium
    D. Coronary sinus

85. Which structure is derived form the right horn of the sinus
    venosus?
    A. Rough part of right atrium
    B. Smooth part of right atrium
    C. Superior vena cava
    D. Fossa ovalis

86. Which cervical inter segmental artery forms the axis artery of
    the upper limb?
    A. Fourth   B. Fifth
    C. Sixth   D. Seventh

87. Which lumbar inter segmental artery forms the axis artery of
    the lower limb?
    A. Second   B. Third
    C. Fourth   D. Fifth

88. All of the following are derivatives of the pharyngeal
    endoderm, EXCEPT:
    A. Thyroid gland   B. Parotid gland
    C. Thymus   D. Lungs

89. Form which structure cortex of the suprarenal gland develops?
    A. Paraxial mesoderm   B. Intermediate mesoderm
    C. Lateral plate mesoderm D. Neural crest cells

90. Form which structure medulla of the suprarenal gland
    develops?
    A. Paraxial mesoderm   B. Intermediate mesoderm
    C. Lateral plate mesoderm D. Neural crest cells

91. Which artery is the derivative of the second aortic arch?
A. Maxillary
B. Lingual
C. Facial
D. Stapedial

92. Form which aortic arch common carotid artery develops?
A. Proximal part of 3rd
B. Distal part of 3rd
C. Proximal part of 4th
D. Distal part of 4th

93. Which left aortic arch forms ductus arteriosus?
A. Proximal part of 4th
B. Distal part of 4th
C. Proximal part of 6th
D. Distal part of 6th

94. The internal ear (otic vesicle) develops form which germ layer?
A. Surface ectoderm
B. Neroectoderm
C. Mesoderm
D. Endoderm

95. In cervical vertebra which one of the following represent true transverse element?
A. Anterior root
B. Posterior root
C. Anterior tubercle
D. Posterior tubercle

96. In cervical vertebra all of the following represent costal elements, EXCEPT:
A. Anterior root
B. Posterior root
C. Anterior tubercle
D. Posterior tubercle

97. Which process of lumbar vertebra represents the costal element?
A. Transverse
B. Accessory
C. Mammillary
D. Superior articular

98. Which is the cephalic end of the primitive neural tube?
A. Genu of corpus callosum
B. Rostrum
C. Lamina terminalis
D. Anterior commissure.

99. From which germ layer tympanic membrane develops?
A. Ectoderm
B. Mesoderm
C. Endoderm
D. All of the above

100. In which month urine formation begins in foetus?
A. Second
B. Third
C. Fourth
D. Fifth

101. From which structure iris of the eye develops?
A. Outer layer optic cup
B. Inner layer of optic cup
C. Optic stalk
D. Marginal region of optic cup

102. **During which weeks of intrauterine life physiological umbilical hernia occurs?**
    A. 3 to 6
    B. 6 to 10
    C. 11 to 14
    D. 15 to 20

103. **What is the cranial limit of notochord?**
    A. Oropharyngeal membrane
    B. Prechordal plate
    C. Septum transversum
    C. Pericardial cavity

104. **All of the following are derivatives of the somite, EXCEPT:**
    A. Sternum
    B. Sacrum
    C. Ribs
    D. Thoracic vertebrae

105. **Inferior vena cave develops from all of the following veins on the right side, EXCEPT:**
    A. Posterior cardinal
    B. Supracardinal
    C. Subcardinal
    D. Inter subcardinal anastomosis

106. **Which one of the following is derivative of the paramesonephric duct in male?**
    A. Prostate
    B. Seminal vesicle
    C. Vas deferns
    D. Appendix of testis

107. **Which one of the following is derivative of the gubernaculum ovary?**
    A. Transverse cervical ligament
    B. Round ligament of uterus
    C. Broad ligament
    D. Suspensory ligament of ovary

108. **From which one of the following muscles of the limb is derived?**
    A. Splanchopleuric mesoderm
    B. Myotome of somites
    C. Branchial mesoderm
    D. *In situ* mesoderm

109. **Sertoli cells are concerned with all of the following functions, EXCEPT:**
    A. Form blood testis barrier inhibiting
    B. Secretion of müllerian factor
    C. Spermiation
    C. Induce meiotic division

110. All of the following form interventricular septum, EXCEPT:
    A. Atrioventricular cushion
    B. Spiral septum
    C. Primitive interventricular septum
    D. Septum spurium

111. Which one of the following cells is mesodermal in origan?
    A. Astrocyte
    B. Oligodendrocyte
    C. Microglia
    D. Ependymal cell

112. All of the following cavities are formed by intra-embryonic coelom, EXCEPT:
    A. Oral
    B. Pleural
    C. Pericardial
    D. Peritoneal

113. All of the following are foetal membranes, EXCEPT:
    A. Amnion
    B. Chorion
    C. Yolk sac
    D. Decidua

114. Neck of the spermatozoa contains which organelle?
    A. Mitochondria
    B. Centriole
    C. Nucleus
    D. Golgi apparatus

115. Middle piece of the spermatozoa contains which organelle?
    A. Mitochondria
    B. Golgi apparatus
    C. Nucleus
    D. Rough endoplasmic reticulum

116. Which one of the following is present in the head of the mature sperm?
    A. Golgi apparatus
    B. Mitochondria
    C. Diploid nucleus
    D. Haploid nucleus

117. Which one of the following prevents dispermy?
    A. Capacitation
    B. Compaction
    C. Decidual reaction
    D. Zona reaction

118. All of the following are the results of fertilization, EXCEPT:
    A. Diploid number of chromosome restored
    B. Chromosomal sex is determined
    C. Disintergration of zona pellucida
    D. Initiation of cleavage

119. Which one of the following is a derivative of the ventral meso-gastrium?
    A. Lesser omentum
    B. Greater omentum
    C. Gastrophrenic ligament
    D. Gastrosplenic ligament

120. **Which one of the following is a derivative of the dorsal mesogastrium?**
    A. Lesser omentum
    B. Greater omentum
    C. Falciform ligament
    D. Coronary ligament

121. **All of the following are derivatives of the ventral mesogastrium, EXCEPT:**
    A. Lesser omentum
    B. Greater omentum
    C. Falciform ligament
    D. Triangular ligament

122. **All of the following are derivatives of the dorsal mesogastrium, EXCEPT:**
    A. Lesser omentum
    B. Greater omentum
    C. Lienorenal ligament
    D. Gastrophrenic ligament

123. **The period of maturation of spermatozoa in the female genital tract is called:**
    A. Compaction
    B. Conception
    C. Condensation
    D. Capacitation

124. **Which ligament is the adult remnant of the left umbilical vein?**
    A. Arteriosum
    B. Venosum
    C. Denticulatum
    D. Teres

125. **In primary oocyte, at which stage the cell division is arrested till the age of puberty?**
    A. Anaphase
    B. Metaphase
    C. Diplotene
    D. Leptotene

126. **Which one of the following forms intra-embryonic mesoderm?**
    A. Notochord
    B. Primitive streak
    C. Amnion
    D. Neural crest

127. **Which part of the pancreas is formed by ventral pancreatic bud?**
    A. Upper half of the head
    B. Body
    C. Uncinate process
    D. Tail

128. **All of the following structures are formed in the second week of intrauterine life, EXCEPT:**
    A. Epiblast
    B. Hypoblast
    C. Yolk sac
    D. Primitive streak

129. All of the following structures are formed in the third week of intrauterine life, EXCEPT:
    A. Neural tube
    B. Notochord
    C. Amnion
    D. Primitive streak

130. All of the following are derivatives of diencephalon, EXCEPT:
    A. Thalamus
    B. Hypothalamus
    C. Anterior pituitary
    D. Posterior pituitary

131. From which one of the following, anterior pituitary develops?
    A. Neuroectoderm
    B. Surface ectoderm
    C. Mesoderm
    D. Endoderm

132. All of the following are derivatives of urogenital sinus, EXCEPT:
    A. Prostate
    B. Bulbourethral glands
    C. Seminal vesicles
    D. Urethra except navicular fossa

133. All of the following are derivatives of the hindgut, EXCEPT:
    A. Urinary bladder
    B. Rectum
    C. Segmoid colon
    D. Ascending colon

134. From which one of the following epithelial reticular cells of the thymus develop?
    A. Surface ectoderm
    B. Neuroectoderm
    C. Mesoderm
    D. Endoderm

135. From which one of the following lymphocytes of the thymus arise?
    A. Surface ectoderm
    B. Neuroectoderm
    C. Mesoderm
    D. Endoderm

136. All of the following structures contribute in the development of the diaphragm, EXCEPT:
    A. Septum transversum
    B. Mesoderm of body wall
    C. Pleuroperitoncal membrane
    D. Ventral mesentery of oesophagus

137. All of the following are derivatives of the septum transversum, EXCEPT:
    A. Central tendon of diaphragm
    B. Fibrous pericardium
    C. Parietal pleura
    D. Kupffer's cells of liver

138. All of the following are derivatives of the urogenital sinus in females, EXCEPT:
    A. Urethra
    B. Paraurethral glands
    C. Vagina
    D. Uterus

139. From which one of the following, posterior pituitary develops?
    A. Neuroectoderm
    B. Surface ectoderm
    C. Mesoderm
    D. Endoderm

140. From which one of the following, olfactory epithelium develops?
    A. Surface ectoderm
    B. Neuroectoderm
    C. Mesoderm
    D. Endoderm

141. Part of which artery is a remnant of first aortic arch?
    A. Facial
    B. Maxillary
    C. Lingual
    D. Stapedial

142. Which artery is a remnant of second aortic arch?
    A. Facial
    B. Maxillary
    C. Lingual
    D. Stapedial

143. Craniopharyngioma is a congenital cystic tumour developing form remanant of which one of the following?
    A. Optic vesicle
    B. Otic vesicle
    C. Evagination of hypothalamus
    D. Rathke's pouch

144. Membranous part of the interventricular septum develops from all of the following, EXCEPT:
    A. Fused atrioventricular cushions
    B. Right bulbar ridge
    C. Left bulbar ridge
    D. Septum spurium

145. Which one of the following germ layer forms membranous labyrinth?
    A. Surface ectoderm
    B. Neuroectoderm
    C. Mesoderm
    D. Endoderm

146. Which one of the following germ layer forms bony labyrinth?
    A. Surface ectoderm
    B. Neuroectoderm
    C. Mesoderm
    D. Endoderm

147. The epiblast is capable of formation of which of the following germ layers?
   A. Ectoderm
   B. Ectoderm and mesoderm
   C. Ectoderm and endoderm
   D. Ectoderm, mesoderm and endoderm

148. In the beginning of which week of embryonic development will a woman experience her first missed menstrual period?
   A. 3rd   B. 4th
   C. 6th   D. 8th

149. From which of the following veins hepatic sinusoids are derived?
   A. Supracardinal   B. Subcardinal
   C. Vitelline   D. Posterior cardinal

150. How soon afterbirth does the foramen ovale close functionally?
   A. Immediately afterbirth   B. 1 to 2 hours
   C. 1 to 2 days   D. 1 to 2 weeks

151. How soon afterbirth ductus arteriosus close functionally?
   A. Immediately afterbirth   B. 1 to 2 hours
   C. 1 to 2 days   D. 1 to 2 weeks

152. At the completion of oogenesis how many mature oocytes are formed from each primary oocyte?
   A. One   B. Two
   C. Three   D. Four

153. Which one of the following establishes anterior/posterior axis in human development?
   A. Premitive streak   B. Notochord
   C. Neural tube   D. Somites

154. Bones of the upper limb develop from which of the following mesoderm?
   A. Paraxial   B. Intermediate
   C. Lateral   D. Extraembryonic

155. Which flexure develops between metencephalon and myelencephalon?
   A. Cephalic   B. Mesencephalic
   C. Pontine   D. Cervical

156. **Bones of the lower limb develop from which of the following mesoderm?**
    A. Paraxial   B. Intermediate
    C. Lateral   D. Extraembryonic

157. **During fourth week of development, at which vertebral level diaphragm is located?**
    A. C3, C4, C5   B. T3,T4,T5
    C. T8, T9, T10   D. L1, L2, L3

158. **During which week of development diaphragm descends to its adult position, i.e. L1 level?**
    A. Sixth   B. Eighth
    C. Tenth   D. Twelfth

159. **During which week of pregnancy first foetal movements (quickening) occur in a pregnant woman?**
    A. 8 to 11   B. 12 to 15
    C. 16 to 20   D. 21 to 24

160. **In the production of female gametes which of the following cells can remain dormant for 12 to 40 years?**
    A. Primordial germ cells   B. Primary oocytes
    C. Secondary oocytes   D. First polar body

161. **In the production of male gametes, which of the following cells remains dormant for 12 years?**
    A. Primordial germ cells   B. Primary spermatocytes
    C. Secondary spermatocytes D. Spermatids

162. **Approximately how many million sperms will be ejaculated by a normal fertile male during sexual intercourse?**
    A. 25   B. 50
    C. 100   D. 350

163. **About how many primary oocytes are ovulated over the entire reproductive life of a woman?**
    A. 480   B. 40,000
    C. 20,0000   D. 70,0000

164. **Inter-maxillary segment is formed by fusion of which prominences?**
    A. Maxillary   B. Mandibular
    C. Lateral nasal   D. Medial nasal

165. **When does the metanephros become functional?**
    A. 4th week of development
    B. 10th week of development

C. Just before birth

D. Just after birth

166. An urachal cyst is a remnant of which of the following structure?

   A. Urogenital sinus   B. Urogenital ridge
   C. Allantois   D. Yolk sac

167. The indifferent embryo begins phenotypic sexual differentiation during which week of development?

   A. Fifth   B. Seventh
   C. Twelfth   D. Twentieth

168. The indifferent embryo completes phenotypic sexual differentiation during which week of development?

   A. Fifth   B. Seventh
   C. Twelfth   D. Twentieth

169. The rostral and caudal neuropores close during which week of embryonic development?

   A. Fourth   B. Sixth
   C. Eighth   D. Tenth

170. Which one of the following, basal ganglion is derived from the diencephalon?

   A. Candate nucleus   B. Globus pallidus
   C. Putamen   D. Amygdaloid body

171. When are the axons of the corticospinal tracts fully myelinated?

   A. Mid foetal period   B. At birth
   C. End of first year   D. End of the second year

172. At the birth the spinal cord ends at which vertebral level?

   A. T12   B. L1
   C. L3   D. S4

173. Which one of the following conditions results from failure of closure of anterior neuropore?

   A. Hydrocephalus   B. Anencephaly
   C. Meningoencephalocele D. Craniosynostosis

174. Which of the following give rise to pancreatic islets?

   A. Surface ectoderm   B. Neuroectoderm
   C. Mesoderm   D. Endoderm

175. Kuffers cells of the liver are derived from which one of the following?

   A. Surface ectoderm   B. Neuroectoderm
   C. Mesoderm   D. Endoderm

176. The lining of the lower part of the anal canal is derived from which one of the following?
    A. Surface ectoderm
    B. Neuroectoderm
    C. Mesoderm
    D. Endoderm

177. In which stage of the lung maturation, the blood-air barrier is established?
    A. Psuedoglandular
    B. Canalicular
    C. Terminal sac
    D. Alveolar

178. How soon afterbirth does the foramen ovale close structurally?
    A. 1 to 2 hours
    B. 1 to 2 weeks
    C. 1 to 3 months
    D. 1 year

179. How soon afterbirth does the ductus arteriosus close structurally?
    A. 1 to 2 hours
    B. 1 to 2 weeks
    C. 1 to 3 months
    D. 1 year

180. Components of the blood-air barrier in the lungs are derived from which of the following sources?
    A. Visceral mesoderm and somatic mesoderm
    B. Visceral mesoderm and ectoderm
    C. Ectoderm and endoderm
    D. Visceral mesoderm and endoderm

181. The proximal part of the aorta is derived from which of the following?
    A. Bulbus cordis
    B. Truncus arteriosus
    C. Primitive ventricle
    D. Primitive atrium

182. The right renal vein is derived from which of the following vein?
    A. Subcardinal
    B. Supracardinal
    C. Vitelline
    D. Mesonephric

183. The superior mesenteric vein is derived from which of the following vein?
    A. Subcardinal
    B. Supracardinal
    C. Umbilical
    D. Vitelline

184. Which of the following is present in the intervillous spaces of the placenta?
    A. Foetal blood
    B. Maternal blood
    C. Foetal and maternal blood
    D. Amniotic fluid

185. Between which two layers, is the extraembronic mesoderm located?
   A. Epiblast and hypoblast
   B. Syncitiotrophoblast and cytotrophablast
   C. Exocoeloric membrane and cytotrophoblast
   D. Exocoelomic membrane and syncitiotrophoblast

186. During second week of development by which of the following means, embryoblast receive their nutrients?
   A. Diffusion   B. Osmosis
   C. Foetal capillaries   D. Yolk sac

187. Which of the following site of future is marked by the prochordal plate?
   A. Umbilical cord   B. Nose
   C. Mouth   D. Heart

188. Which process establishes the three germ layers?
   A. Neurulation   B. Gastrulation
   C. Angiogenesis   D. Lateral folding

189. Formation of which structure is the first indication of gastrulation?
   A. Primitive streak   B. Notochord
   C. Neural tube   D. Tertiary chronic villi

190. Which of the following is derived from the intermediate mesoderm?
   A. Somites   B. Kidneys
   C. Notochord   D. Heart

191. By the end of which week the developing embryo has a distinct human appearance?
   A. Sixth   B. Seventh
   C. Eighth   D. Twelfth

192. Lateral plate mesoderm is divided into two distinct layers by the formation of which of the following?
   A. Extraembryonic coelom   B. Intraembryonic coelom
   C. Notochord   D. Yolk sac

193. What is the normal amount of amniotic fluid in milliliters at term?
   A. 500   B. 1000
   C. 1500   D. 2000

194. How soon after fertilization does the blastocyst begins implantation?

A. 12 hours   B. 1st day
C. 2nd day   D. 6th day

195. Where does the blastocyst normally implant?

A. Functional layer of cervix
B. Functional layer of endometrium
C. Basal layer of endometrium
D. Myometrium

196. Which of the following components plays the most active role in invading the endometrium during blastocyst implantation?

A. Epiblast
B. Hypoblast
C. Syncitiotrophoblast
D. Extraembryonic somatic mesoderm

197. When do the oogonia enter meiosis I and undergo DNA replication to form primary oocytes?

A. During foetal life   B. At birth
C. At puberty   D. During ovulation

198. When does a secondary oocyte complete its second meiotic division to become a mature ovum?

A. Before birth   B. At puberty
C. At ovulation   D. At fertilization

199. Which one of the following is the result of failure of the urethral folds to fuse?

A. Epispadius   B. Hypospadias
C. Cryptorchidism   D. Ectopia vesicae

200. Extraocular muscles develop from which of the following?

A. Preotic myotome   B. Occipital myotome
C. Epimere   D. Hypomere

201. Lateral rotation of upper limbs take place in which weeks of development?

A. 4 to 5   B. 6 to 8
C. 9 to 10   D. 11 to 12

202. Medial rotation of lower limbs take place in which weeks of development?

A. 4 to 5   B. 6 to 8
C. 9 to 10   D. 11 to 12

203. In which direction rotation of upper limbs take place during 6 to 8 weeks of development?

A. Medially 90°

B. Laterally 90°

C. Medially 180°

D. Laterally 180°

204. In which direction rotation of lower limbs take place during 6 to 8 weeks of development?

A. Medially 90°

B. Laterally 90°

C. Medially 180°

D. Laterally 180°

205. Approximately at which day of development first pair of somites appear in the occipital region?

A. 16

B. 20

C. 22

D. 24

206. At which day of development allantois appears in the caudal wall of the yolk sac?

A. 14

B. 16

C. 18

D. 20

207. During spermatogenesis all of the following cells divide, EXCEPT:

A. Spermatogonia

B. Primary oocyte

C. Secondary oocyte

D. Spermatid

208. Which one of the following cells undergoes spermiogenesis?

A. Spermatogonia

B. Primary oocyte

C. Secondary oocyte

D. Spermatid

209. How many spermatids are formed by each differentiating spermatogonium?

A. 64

B. 128

C. 256

D. 512

210. Which one of the following is formed by the outer layer of the optic cup?

A. Sclera

B. Choroid

C. Pigment layer of retina

D. Neural layer of retina

211. Which one of the following is formed by the inner layer of the optic cup?

A. Sclera

B. Choroid

C. Pigment layer of retina

D. Neural layer of retina

212. **Which one of the following structures represents rostral end of the neural tube?**
    A. Genu of corpus callosum
    B. Lamina terminalis
    C. Frontal pole
    D. Paraterminal gyrus

213. **All of the following are derivatives of the neuroectoderm, EXCEPT:**
    A. Retina
    B. Posterior layer of iris
    C. Optic nerve
    D. Lens

214. **Premature closure of foramen of foramen ovale results in:**
    A. Left ventricular hypertrophy
    B. Right ventricular hypertrophy
    C. Underdeveloped right atrium
    D. Pulmonary stenosis

215. **From which one of the following develop basal ganglia?**
    A. Telencephalon
    B. Diancephalon
    C. Metencephalon
    D. Myelencephalon

216. **From which one of the following develop collecting tubules of the kidney?**
    A. Pronephros
    B. Mesonephros
    C. Metanephros
    D. Ureteric bud

217. **Which of the following develops from the endoderm?**
    A. Liver parenchyma
    B. Trigone of the bladder
    C. Cells lining renal tubules
    D. Cells lining fallopian tubes

218. **All of the following are derivatives of the diencephalon, EXCEPT:**
    A. Mammillary bodies
    B. Pineal body
    C. Optic cup
    D. Anterior pituitary

219. **How many microns is the length of a mature human spermatozoon?**
    A. 10 to 20
    B. 50 to 60
    C. 100 to 120
    D. 200

220. **All of the following are derivatives of the mesoderm, EXCEPT:**
    A. Ureter
    B. Uterus
    C. Gall bladder
    D. Epididymis

221. **Which one of the following secrets müllerian inhibiting substance?**
    A. Anterior pituitary
    B. Adrenal cortex
    C. Theca cells
    D. Leydig cells

222. All of the following regions of the hypothalamus are dervatives of the diencephalon, EXCEPT:
   A. Preoptic
   B. Supraoptic
   C. Tuberal
   D. Mammillary

223. Which one of the following anomalies arises due to failure of closure of the cranial end of the neural tube?
   A. Microcephaly
   B. Hydrocephaly
   C. Anencephaly
   D. Meningomyelocele

224. During formation of a vertebra, which one of the following is intersegmental in position?
   A. Intervertebral disc
   B. Artery
   C. Spinal nerve
   D. Myotome

225. Which one of the following has inductive effect on the development of the neural tube?
   A. Primitive node
   B. Primitive streak
   C. Notochord
   D. Prochordal plate

226. What is the characteristics of a baby born to a woman, who has taken thalidomide during her second month of pregnancy?
   A. Syndactyly
   B. Polydactyly
   C. Meromelia
   D. Sirenomelia

227. With which one of the following, amniochorionic membrane fuses, so that amnion obliterates the uterine cavity?
   A. Chorion leave
   B. Decidua basalis
   C. Decidua capsularis
   D. Decidua parietalis

228. What type of placenta is human placenta?
   A. Epitheliochorial
   B. Endothelialchorial
   C. Haemoendothelial
   D. Haemochorial

229. The ascent of the horseshoe kidney is arrested by which one of the following arteries?
   A. Median sacral
   B. Inferior mesenteric
   C. Superior mesenteric
   D. Coeliac axis

230. Doppler foetal heart rate is first audible in which week of pregnancy?
   A. Eighth
   B. Twelfth
   C. Sixteenth
   D. Eighteenth

231. **Which one of the following conditions is indicated by low values of Human Chorionic Gonadotropin (hCG)?**
    A. Ectopic pregnancy
    B. Multiple pregnancy
    C. Hydatidiform mole
    D. Gestational trophoblastic neoplasia

232. **All of the following conditions are indicated by elevated values of human chorionic gonadotropin (hCG), EXCEPT:**
    A. Ectopic pregnancy
    B. Multiple pregnancy
    C. Hydatidiform mole
    D. Gestational trophoblastic neoplasia

233. **Which one of the following conditions is indicated by marked decreased values of serum ± fetoprotein (AFP):**
    A. Anencephaly   B. Spina bifida
    C. Down's syndrome   D. Oesophageal atresia

234. **All of the following conditions are indicated by elevated values of serum α-fetoprotein (AFP), EXCEPT:**
    A. Anencephaly   B. Spina bifida
    C. Down's syndrome   D. Oesophageal atresia

235. **Which genes control the basic segmentation of human embryo in the craniocaudal direction during the embryonic period?**
    A. Hox (homeobox) complex B. Hedgehog
    C. WNT   D. Fibroblast growth factors

236. **Remnants of which of the following, arises sacrococcygeal teratoma?**
    A. Notochord   B. Primitive streak
    C. Neural tube   D. Yolk sac

237. **Which structure is derived from the same embryonic primordium as the kidney?**
    A. Adrenal medulla   B. Liver
    C. Pineal gland   D. Gonads

238. **The left renal vein is derived from all of the following veins, EXCEPT:**
    A. Mesonephric
    B. Posterior cardinal
    C. Intersubcardinal anastomosis
    D. Left subcardinal

239. The suprarenal veins are derived from which of the following veins?
    A. Mesonephric
    B. Posterior cardinal
    C. Supracardinal
    D. Subcardinal

240. The gonadal veins are derived from which of the following veins?
    A. Mesonephric
    B. Posterior cardinal
    C. Supracardinal
    D. Subcardinal

241. The portal vein is derived from which of the following veins?
    A. Umbilical
    B. Vitelline
    C. Supracardinal
    D. Subcardinal

242. All of the following arteries are the derivatives of ventral splanchnic arteries, EXCEPT:
    A. Bronchial
    B. Coronary
    C. Oesophageal
    D. Superior mesenteric

243. All of the following arteries are the derivatives of lateral splanchnic arteries, EXCEPT:
    A. Suprarenal
    B. Phrenic
    C. Testicular
    D. Superior mesenteric

244. Which of the following arteries is the derivative of dorso-lateral arteries?
    A. Phrenic
    B. Lumbar
    C. Suprarenal
    D. Gonadal

245. From which of the following ascending aorta is formed?
    A. Right horn of aortic sac
    B. Left horn of aortic sac
    C. Truncus arteriosus
    D. Dorsal aorta

246. From which of the following pulmonary trunk is formed?
    A. Right horn of aortic sac
    B. Left horn of aortic sac
    C. Truncus arteriosus
    D. Dorsal aorta

247. From which of the following brachiocephalic arteries is formed?
    A. Right horn of aortic sac
    B. Left horn of aortic sac
    C. Truncus arteriosus
    D. Dorsal aorta

248. From which of the following, the choroid plexus of the fourth ventricle is derived?
    A. Alar plate
    B. Floor plate
    C. Roof plate
    D. Rhombic lip

249. From which of the following, pancreatic islets are derived?

    A. Surface ectoderm   B. Neuroectoderm
    C. Mesoderm   D. Endoderm

250. In which period of lung development the blood-air barrier established?

    A. Pseudoglandular   B. Canalicular
    C. Terminal sac   D. Alveolar

251. Pulmonary hypoplasia is commonly associated with which of the following conditions?

    A. Diaphragmatic hernia
    B. Hyaline membrane disease
    C. Tracheo-oesophageal fistula
    D. Congenital bronchial cysts

252. Congenital diaphragmatic hernia is usually life threatening, because it is associated with:

    A. Pulmonary hyperplasia   B. Pulmonary hypoplasia
    C. Liver hypoplasia   D. Liver agenesis

253. Fusion of which of the following prominences forms inter-maximally segment?

    A. Maxillary   B. Mandibular
    C. Lateral nasal   D. Medial nasal

254. Treacher Collins syndrome is associated with which of the pharyngeal arches?

    A. First   B. Second
    C. Third   D. Fourth

255. What structure would most likely be involved in Treacher Collins syndrome?

    A. Thyroid gland   B. Malleus
    C. Stapes   D. Hyoid bone

256. In which week of development, does the metanephros becomes functional?

    A. Third   B. Fourth
    C. Tenth   D. Fourteenth

257. A urachal cyst is a remnant of which of the following?

    A. Urogenital sinus   B. Cloaca
    C. Mesonphric duct   D. Allantois

258. From which of the following podocytes of Bowman's capsule are derived?
    A. Ectoderm
    B. Mesoderm
    C. Endoderm
    D. Neural crest cells

259. From which of the following transitional epithelium of the urinary bladder is derived?
    A. Ectoderm
    B. Mesoderm
    C. Endoderm
    D. Neural crest cells

260. From which of the following transitional epithelium of the ureter is derived?
    A. Ectoderm
    B. Mesoderm
    C. Endoderm
    D. Neural crest cells

261. The proximal convoluted tubules of the adult kidney are derived from which of the following?
    A. Ureteric bud
    B. Metanephric vesicle
    C. Mesonephric duct
    D. Mesonephric tubules

262. Scaphocephaly is caused by premature closure of which of the following sutures?
    A. Sagittal
    B. Coronal
    C. Lmbdoid
    D. Sphenoparietal

263. Brachycephaly is caused by premature closure of which of the following sutures?
    A. Sagittal
    B. Coronal
    C. Lambdoid
    D. Sphenoparietal

264. In which of the following conditions pedicles of the vertebral arch fail to fuse with the vertebral body?
    A. Cleft vertebra
    B. Block vertebra
    C. Hemivertebra
    D. Spondylesthesis

265. Bilateral cryptorchidisim usually results in:
    A. Testicular feminization syndrome
    B. Male pseudo-intersexuality
    C. Impontence
    D. Sterility

266. A newborn baby boy has a tuft of hair on his back in the lumbar region. Which of the following is the most likely diagnosis?
    A. Spondylesthesis
    B. Block vertebra
    C. Spina bifida occulta
    D. Brevicollis

Histology

1. **All of the following cells are multinucleated, EXCEPT:**
   A. Osteoclasts
   B. Skeletal myocytes
   C. Cytotrophoblasts
   D. Syncytiotrophoblasts

2. **Which fibres are present in the loose areolar tissue?**
   A. Collagen
   B. Elastic
   C. Reticular
   D. All of the above

3. **In which one of the following hyaline cartilage is present?**
   A. Menisci
   B. Head of femur
   C. Labrum glenoidale
   D. Labrum acetabulum

4. **Which cells of the testis form the blood-testis barrier?**
   A. Sustentacular (Sertoli)
   B. Interstitial cells of Leydig
   C. Spermatogonia
   D. Primary spermatocytes

5. **Which cell organelle provides energy to various cellular functions?**
   A. Golgi apparatus
   B. Lysosomes
   C. Mitochondria
   D. Centriole

6. **In all of the following taste buds are present, EXCEPT:**
   A. Filiform papillae
   B. Fungiform papillae
   C. Circumvallate papillae
   D. Epiglottis

7. **In which one of the following Brunner's glands are present?**
   A. Duodenum
   B. Jejunum
   C. Ileum
   D. Stomach

8. **Which cell forms myelin sheath in peripheral nerves?**
   A. Oligodendrocytes
   B. Fibroblasts
   C. Satellite cells
   D. Schwann cells

9. **Which organelle is involved in intracellular digestion?**
   A. Mitochondria
   B. Golgi apparatus
   C. Lysosome
   D. Rough endoplasmic reticulum

10. Junctional complex includes all of the following, EXCEPT:
- A. Zonula occludens
- B. Zonula adherens
- C. Desmosome
- D. Gap junction

11. All of the following are simple epithelia, EXCEPT:
- A. Transitional
- B. Neuroepithelial cells
- C. Myoepithelial cells
- D. Pseudostratified epithelium

12. Which fibres are present in tendon?
- A. Collagen
- B. Reticular
- C. Elastic
- D. All of the above

13. In which pars of the pituitary gland pituicytes are present?
- A. Distalis
- B. Intermedia
- C. Tuberalis
- D. Nervosa

14. Intervertebral discs are made up of which type of tissue?
- A. Fibrous tissue
- B. White fibrocartilage
- C. Hyaline cartilage
- D. Elastic cartilage

15. In which organelle transcription of protein takes place?
- A. Nucleus
- B. Golgi apparatus
- C. Ribosomes
- D. Rough endoplasmic reticulum

16. In which one of the following goblet cells are absent?
- A. Stomach
- B. Duodenum
- C. Appendix
- D. Rectum

17. All of the following are white fibrocartilages, EXCEPT:
- A. Intervertibral disc
- B. Interpubic disc
- C. Tracheal rings
- D. Mensci of the knee joint

18. What type of epithelium is urothelium?
- A. Squamous
- B. Cuboidal
- C. Transitional
- D. Pseudostratified

19. In which one of the following lymphatic nodules are absent?
- A. Spleen
- B. Thymus
- C. Tonsil
- D. Lymph node

20. Which one of the following is an example of dense irregular connective tissue?
- A. Dermis
- B. Bone
- C. Adipose
- D. Tendon

21. In which blood vessel internal elastic lamina is very prominent?
    - A. Large sized artery
    - B. Medium sized artery
    - C. Large sized vein
    - D. Medium sized vein

22. In which of the following oxyntic cells are present?
    - A. Stomach
    - B. Thyroid
    - C. Parathyroid
    - D. Pituitary

23. What type of gland is kidney?
    - A. Simple tubular
    - B. Compound tubular
    - C. Compound alveolar
    - D. Compound tubulo-alveolar

24. Menisci are made up of which type of tissue?
    - A. Fibrous tissue
    - B. White fibrocartilage
    - C. Elastic cartilage
    - D. Articular cartilage

25. What is the lining epithelium of thin segment of loop of Henle?
    - A. Simple columnar
    - B. Simple squamous
    - C. Simple cuboidal
    - D. Stratified squamous

26. All of the following are characteristics of skeletal muscle, EXCEPT:
    - A. Cylindrical cells
    - B. Syncitium
    - C. Striations
    - D. Nuclei peripherally placed

27. What type of epithelium is anterior epithelium of the cornea?
    - A. Pseudostratified
    - B. Transitional
    - C. Stratified cuboidal
    - D. Stratified squamous non-keratinized

28. Cardiac muscle is able to function as a syncytium because of which structure?
    - A. Branching fibres
    - B. Intercalated disc
    - C. Desmosomes
    - D. Gap-junctions

29. Which is the largest organelle in eukaryote?
    - A. Endoplasmic reticulum
    - B. Nucleus
    - C. Cytoskeleton
    - D. Golgi body

30. In which one of the following Haversian system is present?
    - A. Cortical bone
    - B. Cancellous bone
    - C. Teeth
    - D. Cartilage

31. In which one of the following myenteric plexus is present?
   A. Large intestine
   B. Esophagus
   C. Stomach
   D. All of the above

32. Which one of the following is lined by transitional epithelium?
   A. Epididymis
   B. Penile urethra
   C. Ureter
   D. Colon

33. Which epithelium lines parietal peritoneum?
   A. Simple squqmous
   B. Stratified squamous
   C. Simple cuboidal
   D. Simple columnar

34. In central nervous system myelin sheath is formed by which cells?
   A. Oligodendrocytes
   B. Microglia
   C. Schwann cells
   D. Astrocytes

35. In which organ Kupffer's cells are present?
   A. Spleen
   B. Bone marrow
   C. Liver
   D. Adrenal

36. The ureter is lined by which epithelium?
   A. Stratifed squamous
   B. Cuboidal
   C. Cilliated columanar
   D. Transitional

37. Which one of the following glands is holocrine?
   A. Salivary
   B. Mammary
   C. Sebaceous
   D. Gastric

38. In which one of the following juxta-glomerular cells are present?
   A. Proximal convoluted tubule
   B. Distal convoluted tubule
   C. Smooth muscular cells of afferent arteriole
   D. Smooth muscular cells of efferent arteriole

39. In which gland ducts of Bellini are present?
   A. Pancreas
   B. Parotid
   C. Kidney
   D. Liver

40. In which one of the following space of Disse is present?
   A. Spleen
   B. Lymph node
   C. Liver
   D. Bone

41. In which one of the following macula densa is present?
- A. Proximal convoluted tubule
- B. Distal convoluted tubule
- C. Smooth muscular cells of afferent arteriole
- D. Smooth muscular cells of efferent arteriole

42. Which gland is both apocrine and merocrine?
- A. Salivary
- B. Sweat
- C. Mammary
- D. Gastric

43. In the wall of which blood vessel vasa vasorum are more extensive?
- A. Vein
- B. Elastic artery
- C. Muscular artery
- D. Arteriole

44. Which one of the following structures is surrounded by pericytes?
- A. Capillary
- B. Elastic artery
- C. Muscular artery
- D. Arteriole

45. The sinusoidal capillaries are found in all of the following, EXCEPT:
- A. Kidney
- B. Liver
- C. Spleen
- D. Bone marrow

46. In which organ fenestrated capillaries is present?
- A. Kidney
- B. Liver
- C. Spleen
- D. Bone marrow

47. What type of neurons is present in autonomic ganglia?
- A. Unipolar
- B. Pseudounipolar
- C. Bipolar
- D. Multipolar

48. What type of neurons is present in dorsal root ganglia?
- A. Unipolar
- B. Pseudounipolar
- C. Bipolar
- D. Multipolar

49. Parafollicular cells are present in which gland?
- A. Parathyroid
- B. Thyroid
- C. Pituitary
- D. Mammary

50. In which of the following oxyphil cells is present?
- A. Stomach
- B. Thyroid
- C. Parathyroid
- D. Pituitary

51. Which one of the following forms the blood-testis barrier?
  A. Tunica albuginea B. Tunica vasculosa
  C. Tunica vaginalis D. Sertoli cells

52. In which one of the following stereocilia is present?
  A. Trachea B. Small intestine
  C. Ductus epididymis D. Fallopian tube

53. At the time of ovulation which cell is liberated?
  A. Oogonium B. Primary oocyte
  C. Secondary oocyte D. Ovun

54. White mater of the nervous system contains all of the following, EXCEPT:
  A. Myelinated axons B. Nonmyelinated axons
  C. Dendrites D. Neuroglia

55. In which one of the following mesangial cells is present?
  A. Skin B. kidney
  C. Lungs D. Small intestine

56. In which one of the following Paneth cells is present?
  A. Small intestine B. Large intestine
  C. Stomach D. Oesophagus

57. Superficial cells of which lining epithelium show unique thickened regions-plaques?
  A. Pseudostratified B. Stratified squamous
  C. Stratified columan D. Transitional

58. All of the following cells of anterior pituitary are basophils, EXCEPT:
  A. Thyrotrophs B. Somatotrophs
  C. Gonadotrophs D. Corticotrophs

59. Which cells of the anterior pituitary are acidophils?
  A. Thyrotrophs B. Somatotrophs
  C. Gonadotrophs D. Corticotrophs

60. Herring bodies are present in which part of the pituitary gland?
  A. Distalis B. Nervosa
  C. Tuberalis D. Intermedia

61. Testis has following tunics, EXCEPT:
  A. Adventitia B. Vasculosa
  C. Albuginea D. Vaginalis

62. What type of epithelium is present in ductus epididymis?
- A. Simple columnar
- B. Transitional
- C. Stratified columnar
- D. Psuedostratified columnar

63. Tunica albuginea is present in all of the following, EXCEPT:
- A. Penis
- B. Epididymis
- C. Testis
- D. Ovary

64. What is the life of span of corpus luteum of pregnancy?
- A. 10 to 12 days
- B. 4 to 5 weeks
- C. 4 to 5 months
- D. 9 months

65. In which one of the following Bowman's glands is present?
- A. Duodenum
- B. Oesophagus
- C. Olfactory mucosa
- D. Kidney

66. Fibromuscular stroma is the characteristics of which gland?
- A. Thyroid
- B. Prostate
- C. Testis
- D. Mammary

67. Amyloid bodies are present in which gland?
- A. Thyroid
- B. Prostate
- C. Parathyroid
- D. Pancreas

68. Von Ebner's glands are present in which one of the following?
- A. Duodenum
- B. Tongue
- C. Eyelid
- D. Trachea

69. Which cells are present in neurohypophysis?
- A. Acidophils
- B. Basophils
- C. Chromophils
- D. Pituicytes

70. All of the following cells are present in the anterior pituitary, EXCEPT:
- A. Acidophills
- B. Basophills
- C. Chromophills
- D. Pituicytes

71. All of the following cells are present in the inner nuclear layer of the retina, EXCEPT:
- A. Ganglion
- B. Bipolar
- C. Amacrine
- D. Horizontal

72. What type of gland is sebaceous gland?
- A. Merocrine
- B. Apocrine
- C. Holocrine
- D. Paracrine

73. What type of gland is tarsal gland?
   A. Branched alveolar
   B. Compound alveolar
   C. Compound tubuloalveolar
   D. Branched tubular

74. Which epithelium lines the surface of the endometrium?
   A. Simple squamous
   B. Simple cuboidal
   C. Simple columnar
   D. Psuedo-stratified columnar

75. Which one of the following cells is present in all mature follicles before ovulation?
   A. Oogonium
   B. Primary oocyte
   C. Secondary oocyte
   D. Ovum

76. All of the following are antigen presenting cells, EXCEPT:
   A. Langerhan
   B. Kupffer
   C. Macrophage
   D. Merckel

77. Apocrine sweat glands are found in the deep dermis of all of the following regions, EXCEPT:
   A. Axilla
   B. Anus
   C. Palm
   D. Areola of breast

78. Goblet cells are present in all of the following, EXCEPT:
   A. Stomach
   B. Small intestine
   C. Large intestine
   D. Trachea

79. Which cells cover Peyer's patches?
   A. Paneth
   B. M
   C. Clara
   D. Mesangial

80. In which one of the following dust cells is present?
   A. Bronchiole
   B. Terminal bronchiole
   C. Respiratory bronchiole
   D. Alveoli

81. In which part of respiratory tract Clara cells is present?
   A. Trachea
   B. Bronchus
   C. Bronchiole
   D. Alveoli

82. In which one of the following Leydig's cells is present?
   A. Kidney
   B. Ovary
   C. Testis
   D. Liver

83. Centroacinar cells are present in the acini of which gland?
   A. Parotid
   B. Submandibular
   C. Mammary
   D. Pancreas

84. **What type of tubular gland is sweat gland?**
    A. Simple
    B. Simple coiled
    C. Branched
    D. Compound

85. **Which one of the following cells of connective tissue is a wandering cell?**
    A. Fat
    B. Plasma
    C. Fibroblast
    D. Pigment

86. **Which one of the following cells of connective tissue is a fixed cell?**
    A. Plasma
    B. Mast
    C. Fat
    D. Lymphocyte

87. **What type of glands is crypt of Lieberkühn?**
    A. Simple tubular
    B. Simple coiled tubular
    C. Branched alveolar
    D. Branched tubular

88. **What type of glands is Brunner's gland?**
    A. Simple tubular
    B. Simple alveolar
    C. Compound tubular
    D. Compound alveolar

89. **What type of epithelium is present in the conjunctiva?**
    A. Simple cuboidal
    B. Simple columnar
    C. Stratified cuboidal
    D. Stratified columnar

90. **What type of epithelium is present in the sweat glands?**
    A. Simple cuboidal
    B. Simple sqamous
    C. Stratified cuboidal
    D. Stratified columnar

91. **In all of the following endocrine glands secretory units are present in the form of cords, EXCEPT:**
    A. Thyroid
    B. Parathyroid
    C. Anterior pituitary
    D. Adrenal medulla

92. **Myoepithelial cells are present in all of the following glands, EXCEPT:**
    A. Mammary
    B. Lacrimal
    C. Salivary
    D. Sebaceous

93. **The gray matter of cerebellum consists of all of the following layers, EXCEPT**
    A. Molecular
    B. Multiform
    C. Purkinjee cell
    D. Granular

94. In which part of the tooth, interglobular spaces are present?
- A. Enamel
- B. Cementum
- C. Dentinoenamel junction
- D. Dentinal cementum junction

95. Which cells produce enamel of the tooth?
- A. Chondroblast
- B. Cementocyte
- C. Odontoblast
- D. Ameloblast

96. Which cells produce dentin of the tooth?
- A. Chondroblast
- B. Cementocyte
- C. Odontoblast
- D. Ameloblast

97. Which one of the following contains organ of Corti?
- A. Saccule
- B. Scala tympani
- C. Scala media
- D. Scala vestibuli

98. Inner and outer limiting membranes of the retina are formed by processes of which cell?
- A. Bipolar
- B. Muller
- C. Amacrine
- D. Horizontal

99. Axons of which cell form optic nerve fibres?
- A. Muller
- B. Rods
- C. Ganglion
- D. Bipolar

100. In which one of the following podocytes is present?
- A. Glomerulus
- B. Proximal convoluted tubule
- C. Visceral layer of Bowman's capsule
- D. Parietal layer of Bowman's

101. In which endocrine gland secretory units are present in the form of follicles?
- A. Thyroid
- B. Parathyroid
- C. Anterior pituitary
- D. Adrenal medulla

102. Which of the following represents intercalated disc of cardiac muscle?
- A. A Band
- B. M line
- C. H zone
- D. Z line

103. Which fibres are formed by fibroblasts?
- A. Collagen
- B. Elastic
- C. Reticular
- D. All of the following

104. Eccentrically placed cartwheel pattern of the nucleus is characteristic of which cells?
- A. Mast
- B. Plasma
- C. Fibroblast
- D. Macrophage

105. Granular cytoplasm is the characteristic of which cell?
A. Plasma
B. Fibroblast
C. Mast
D. Macrophage

106. All of the following are stratified epithelia, EXCEPT:
A. Stratified squamous
B. Stratified columnar
C. Psuedostratified
D. Seminiferous

107. All of the following contain microtubules, EXCEPT:
A. Microvilli
B. Cilia
C. Centriole
D. Flagellum

108. Which cell organelle is concerned with steroid synthesis?
A. Smooth endoplasmic reticulum
B. Rough endoplasmic reticulum
C. Lysosome
D. Mitochondrium

109. All of the following form cytoskeleton, EXCEPT:
A. Microtubules
B. Elastic fibres
C. Intermediate filaments
D. Microfilaments

110. Afferent and efferent lymphatics are present in which one of the following?
A. Thymus
B. Lymph node
C. Spleen
D. Tonsil

111. Which one of the following lymphoid organ is lobulated?
A. Thymus
B. Lymph node
C. Spleen
D. Tonsil

112. In which one of the following lymphoid organ penicillar arteries are present?
A. Thymus
B. Lymph node
C. Spleen
D. Tonsil

113. What type of connecting tissue is present in the umbilical cord?
A. Loose oreolar
B. Dense irregular
C. Reticular
D. Mucoid

114. In which stratum of the epidermis melanocytes are present?
A. Basale
B. Spinosum
C. Granulosum
D. Lucidum

115. Which cells are present in the outer nuclear layer of the retina?
A. Bipolar
B. Ganglion
C. Amcrine
D. Rods and cones

116. **Which fibres are present in the sclera?**
    A. Collagen
    B. Elastic
    C. Reticular
    D. None of the above

117. **Which one of the following lymphoid organs has rich blood supply?**
    A. Thymus
    B. Lymph node
    C. Spleen
    D. Tonsil

118. **Which one of the following Hassal's corpuscles is present?**
    A. Thymus
    B. Lymph node
    C. Spleen
    D. Tonsil

119. **Which one of the following is lymphoepithelial organ?**
    A. Thymus
    B. Lymph node
    C. Spleen
    D. Tonsil

120. **Which is the thymus dependent zone of a lymph node?**
    A. Cortex
    B. Paracortex
    C. Medullary cords
    D. Medullary sinuses

121. **The gray matter of cerebrum contains of all of the following cells, EXCEPT:**
    A. Pyramidial
    B. Fusiform
    C. Purkinjee
    D. Martinoti

122. **In which ducts of salivary glands, isotonic primary saliva is converted into hypotonic saliva by secreting and absorbing certain ions?**
    A. Intercalated
    B. Striated
    C. Intralobular
    D. Interlobular

123. **All of the following cells in the retina are neurons, EXPECT:**
    A. Bipolar
    B. Muller
    C. Amacrine
    D. Horizontal

124. **Which one of the following epithelia lines the mucosa of the oesophagus?**
    A. Stratified columnar
    B. Stratified cuboid
    C. Stratified squamous non-keratinized
    D. Stratified squamous keratinized

125. **All of the following glands have striated ducts, EXCEPT:**
    A. Parotid
    B. Pancreas
    C. Mammary
    D. Submandibular

126. **Centroacinar cells are present in the acini of which one of the following glands?**
    A. Submandibular   B. Mammary
    C. Parotid   D. Pancreas

127. **A cell which does not divide is arrested in which phase of cell cycle?**
    A. S   B. G1
    C. G2   D. G0

128. **Which one of the following connective cells is active in tissue healing?**
    A. Mast cell   B. Myofibroblast
    C. Leucocyte   D. Plasma cell

129. **Which one of the following represent the prickles that are characteristics of keratinocytes in the stratun spinosum?**
    A. Zonula ocludens   B. Zonula adherens
    C. Gap junctions   D. Desmosomes

130. **Which cell migrates into epidermis during embryonic life and may turn into skin cancer?**
    A. Keratinocyte   B. Merckel cell
    C. Langerhan's cell D. Melanocyte

131. **What is the surface modification seen in the epithelial cells of the epididymis?**
    A. Cilia   B. Stereocilia
    C. Microvilli   D. Ruffled border

132. **Celiac disease (sprue) is due to loss of which one of the following?**
    A. Cilia   B. Microvilli
    C. Stereocilia   D. None of the above

133. **From which one of the following lipofuscin pigment in ageing neurons is derived?**
    A. Nissl granules   B. Lysosome
    C. Neurofibrils   D. Golgi apparatus

134. **By which one of the following process, osteoclasts are formed?**
    A. Karyokinesis without cytokinesis
    B. Cytokinesis without karyokinesis
    C. Cytokinesis and karyokinesis
    D. Apopotosis

135. T tubules in the skeletal muscle is a part of which one of the following?
   A. Rough endoplasmic reticulum
   B. Smooth endoplasmic reticulum
   C. Myofilaments
   D. Sarcolemma

136. The sarcoplasmic reticulum in the skeletal muscle is a part of which one of the following?
   A. Rough endoplasmic reticulum
   B. Smooth endoplasmic reticulum
   C. Myofilaments
   D. Sarcolemma

137. What type of stroma is present in the mammary gland?
   A. Fibromuscular
   B. Fibrofatty
   C. Reticular
   D. Fibroelastic

138. What type of stroma is present in the prostate gland?
   A. Fibromuscular
   B. Fibrofatty
   C. Reticular
   D. Fibroelastic

139. Mucoid connective tissue is present postnatally at all of the following sites, EXCEPT:
   A. Umbilical cord
   B. Pulp of the developing tooth
   C. Vitreous humour
   D. Nucleus pulposus

140. All of the following are single contracticle cells, EXCEPT:
   A. Myoepithelial
   B. Myofibroblast
   C. Myoid
   D. Myeloid

141. In the renal cortex, all of the following are present, EXCEPT:
   A. Proximal convoluted tubule
   B. Distal convoluted tubule
   C. Bowman's capsule
   D. Hair pin bend of loop of Henle

142. In which of the following microtubules is absent?
   A. Microvilli
   B. Cilia
   C. Flagella
   D. Centrioles

143. In which of the following microfilaments is present?
   A. Microvilli
   B. Cilia
   C. Flagella
   D. Centrioles

144. **At which stage of cell division mitotic spindle dissociate?**
    A. Prophase
    B. Metaphase
    C. Anaphase
    D. Telophase

145. **At which stage of meiosis I crossing over of chromosomes take place?**
    A. Leptotene
    B. Zygotene
    C. Pachytene
    D. Diplotene

146. **At which stage of meiosis I pairing of chromosomes take place?**
    A. Leptotene
    B. Zygotene
    C. Pachytene
    D. Diplotene

147. **Which one of the following cells shows signet ring appearance?**
    A. Plasma
    B. Fibroblast
    C. Mast
    D. Adipose

148. **Which one of the following cells is elongated with cytoplasmic projections?**
    A. Plasma
    B. Fibroblast
    C. Mast
    D. Adipose

149. **In which of the following precapillary sphincters is present?**
    A. Arteriole
    B. Terminal arteriole
    C. Metaarteriole
    D. Venule

150. **Which one of the following lymphoid organs has both afferent and efferent lymphatics?**
    A. Lymph node
    B. Tonsil
    C. Spleen
    D. Thymus

151. **Which one of the following cells is known as heart failure cell?**
    A. Pneumocyte type I
    B. Pneumocyte type II
    C. Clara cell
    D. Macrophage

152. **In wich of the following glands has serous demilunes?**
    A. Submandibular
    B. Parotid
    C. Sebaceous
    D. Pancreas

153. **In which of the following organs has both skeletal and smooth muscles in the muscularis externa?**
    A. Oesophagus
    B. Stomach
    C. Small intestine
    D. Large instenine

154. Stereocilia are present in all of the following, EXCEPT:
- A. Fallopian tube
- B. Vas deferens
- C. Epididymis
- D. Organ of Corti

155. In which of the following Ito cells is present?
- A. Pancreas
- B. Liver
- C. Organ of Corti
- D. Epidermis

156. In which of the following Paneth cells is present?
- A. Large instenine
- B. Small intestine
- C. Pancreas
- D. Parathyroid

157. In which phase of mitosis nucleolus disappears?
- A. Prophase
- B. Metaphase
- C. Anaphase
- D. Telophase

158. In which phase of mitosis nucleolus reappears?
- A. Prophase
- B. Metaphase
- C. Anaphase
- D. Telophase

159. All of the following are cytoplasmic inclusions, EXCEPT:
- A. Fat droplets
- B. Zymogen granules
- C. Glycogen granules
- D. Lipofuscin granules

160. All of the following form mucus membrane, EXCEPT:
- A. Epithelium
- B. Lamina propria
- C. Muscularis mucosa
- D. Muscularis externa

161. What type of cartilage is present in the bronchi?
- A. Hyaline
- B. Elastic
- C. Fibrocartilage
- D. Articular

162. Capillaries present in the following organs are fenestrated with diaphragm, EXCEPT:
- A. Kideny
- B. Pancreas
- C. Pituitary
- D. Intestinal villi

163. In which of the following organs, capillaries are fenestrated without diaphragm?
- A. Kideny
- B. Pancreas
- C. Pituitary
- D. Intestinal villi

164. Approximately how many layers of collagen bundles are present in the corneal stroma?
- A. 40
- B. 60
- C. 80
- D. 100

165. In which of the following macula densa is present?
- A. Afferent arteriole
- B. Efferent arteriole
- C. Proximal convoluted tubule
- D. Distal convoluted tubule

166. In which of the following juxta-glomerular cells is present?
- A. Afferent arteriole
- B. Efferent arteriole
- C. PCT proximal convoluted tubule
- D. Distal convoluted tubule

167. Aproximately how many seminiferous tubules are present in each testis?
- A. 100–200
- B. 500–1000
- C. 5000–6000
- D. 10,000

168. Primary oocyte completes its first meiotic division at the time of:
- A. Ovulation
- B. Fertilization
- C. Before birth
- D. Puberty

169. Secondary oocyte completes its second division at the time of:
- A. Ovulation
- B. Fertilization
- C. Before birth
- D. Puberty

170. How many micorns are the length of a human spermatozoon?
- A. 10–20
- B. 50–60
- C. 100–200
- D. 300–500

171. What type of ganglia is present in the submucosal and myenteric plexuses of intestine?
- A. Sensory
- B. Sympathetic
- C. Parasympathetic
- D. All of the above

172. In which one of the following conditions reduced bone mineral density is seen?
- A. Osteogenesis imperfecta
- B. Osteoporosis
- C. Osteopetrosis
- D. Osteomalacia

173. Which one of the following conditions is characterized by dense heavy bones (marble bones)?
- A. Osteogenesis imperfecta
- B. Osteoporosis
- C. Osteopetrosis
- D. Osteomalacia

174. Which one of the following conditions is due to calcium deficiency?
A. Osteogenesis imperfecta   B. Osteoporosis
C. Osteopetrosis   D. Osteomalacia

175. Which one of the following conditions is due to deficient amount of type I collagen production?
A. Osteogenesis imperfecta   B. Osteoporosis
C. Osteopetrosis   D. Osteomalacia

176. All of the following cells belong to mononuclear phagocyte system, EXCEPT:
A. Kupffer cells   B. Microglia
C. Osteoclasts   D. Merckel cells

177. How many micrometers are the diameter of an arteriole?
A. 50–100   B. 200–250
C. 300–400   D. 500–600

178. Which of the following layers of an artery are supplied by vasa vasorum?
A. Tunica media and tunica intima
B. Tunica adventitia and tunica media
C. Tunica adventitia and outer part of tunica media
D. All layers of the artery

179. Which of the following epithelium lines the tunica intima of a blood vessel?
A. Simple squamous   B. Simple cuboidal
C. Stratified squamous   D. Pseudostratified columnar

180. Which one of the following ligaments is mainly elastic?
A. Ligamentum patellae   B. Ligamentum flavum
C. Stylomandibular   D. Deltoid

181. Apical surfaces of the luminal cells of which one of the following epithelia show dense plaques?
A. Stratified squamous   B. Stratified cuboid
C. Stratified columnar   D. Transitional

182. With which one of the following pericytes is associated?
A. Alveoli of parotid gland
B. Alveoli of sweat glands
C. Alveoli of mammary gland
D. Capillaries

183. Which one of the following represents the prickles of the keratinocytes of stratum spinosum of the epidermis?

A. Zona occludens
B. Zona adherens
C. Desmosomes
D. Hemidesmosomes

184. Which one of the following connective tissues is present in the papillary layer of the epidermis?

A. Loose areolar
B. Dense regular
C. Dense irregular
D. Adipose

185. Which one of the following connective tissues is present in the reticular layer of the epidermis?

A. Loose areolar
B. Dense regular
C. Dense irregular
D. Adipose

186. In which one of the following structural protein laminin is found?

A. Nuclear membrane
B. Cell membrane
C. Basal lamina of basement membrane
D. Reticular lamina of basement membrane

187. Which one of the following structural components is responsible for the tensile strength of the bone?

A. Calcium hydroxyapatite
B. Osteonectin
C. Collagen type I
D. Collagen type II

188. Which structure is continuous with rough endoplasmic reticulum?

A. Nucleolus
B. Outer nuclear membrane
C. Heterochromatin
D. Euchromatin

189. Which of the following organelles, divides by fission?

A. Peroxisome
B. Golgi apparatus
C. Smooth endoplasmic reticulum
D. Rough endoplasmic reticulum

190. Which one of the following is present in the basement membrane and manufactured by connective cells?

A. Fibrillin
B. Fibronectin
C. Elastin
D. Laminin

Genetics

1. What type of chromosome is Y chromosome?
    A. Acrocentric   B. Metacentric
    C. Submetacentric   D. Telocentric

2. What type of chromosome is first chromosome?
    A. Acrocentric   B. Metacentric
    C. Submetacentric   D. Telocentric

3. What type of chromosome is X chromosome?
    A. Acrocentric   B. Metacentric
    C. Submetacentric   D. Telocentric

4. At which stage of mitosis colchicines stops mitosis?
    A. Prophase   B. Metaphase
    C. Anaphase   D. Telophase

5. What type of genetic disorder is Down's syndrome?
    A. Single gene   B. Chromosomal
    C. Multifactorial   D. All of the above

6. What type of genetic disorder is Phenylketonuria?
    A. Single gene   B. Chromosomal
    C. Multifactorial   D. None of the above

7. What type of disorder is cleft lip?
    A. Single gene   B. Chromosomal
    C. Multifactorial   D. None of the above

8. What type of inheritance is seen in Hairy pinna?
    A. Autosomal dominant   B. Autosomal recessive
    C. Y linked   D. X linked dominant

9. What type of inheritance is seen in dentinogenesis imperfecta?
    A. Autosomal dominant   B. Autosomal recessive
    C. X linked recessive   D. X linked dominant

10. **What type of inheritance is seen in phenylketonuria?**
    A. Autosomal dominant   B. Autosomal recessive
    C. X linked recessive   D. X linked dominant

11. **What type of inheritance is seen in haemophillia?**
    A. Autosomal dominant   B. Autosomal recessive
    C. X linked recessive   D. X linked dominant

12. **What type of inheritance is seen in vitamin D resistant rickets?**
    A. Autosomal dominant   B. Autosomal recessive
    C. X linked recessive   D. X linked dominant

13. **What type of inheritance is seen in partial colour blindness?**
    A. Autosomal dominant   B. Autosomal recessive
    C. X linked recessive   D. X linked dominant

14. **What type of inheritance is seen achondroplasia?**
    A. Autosomal dominant   B. Autosomal recessive
    C. X linked recessive   D. X linked dominant

15. **Which one of the following is the karyotype of Down's syndrome?**
    A. Trisomy 13   B. Trisomy 18
    C. Monosomy 21   D. Trisomy 21

16. **Which one of the following is the karyotype of Turner's syndrome?**
    A. 46 XY   B. 47 XXY
    C. 45 XO   D. 47 XXX

17. **All of the following are clinical features of Down's syndrome, EXCEPT:**
    A. Intelligent quotient 25–50   B. Tall and eunuchoid
    C. Hypotonia   D. Epicanthal folds

18. **All of the following are clinical features of Turner's syndrome, EXCEPT:**
    A. Webbing of neck   B. Cubitus valgus
    C. Epicanthal folds   D. Short stature

19. **Which one of the following is the feature of Klinefelter's syndrome?**
    A. Short stature
    B. Absence of spermatogenesis
    C. Protruding tongue
    D. Cubitus valgus

20. What is the role of colchine in karyotyping?

A. Nourishing medium
B. Antimitotic agent
C. Mitogenic agent
D. Anticoagulant

21. What is the role of foetal calf serum in Karyotyping?

A. Nourishing medium
B. Antimitotic agent
C. Mitogenic agent
D. Anticoagulant

22. What is the role of phytohaemagglutinin in karyotyping?

A. Nourishing medium
B. Antimitotic agent
C. Mitogenic agent
D. Anticoagulant

23. Which one of the following is noninvasive tool in prenatal diagnosis?

A. Amniocentesis
B. Ultrasonography
C. CT scan
D. Chorion villous sampling

24. Which one of the following is a numerical chromosomal aberration?

A. Translocation
B. Tetraploidy
C. Isochromosome
D. Duplication

25. Which one of the following is a structural chromosomal aberration?

A. Translocation
B. Tetraploidy
C. Trisomy
D. Triploidy

26. Chorion villous biopsy is undertaken between which weeks of pregnancy?

A. 4 to 6
B. 8 to 10
C. 14 to 16
D. 20 to 22

27. Amniocentesis is done between which weeks of pregnancy?

A. 8 to 10
B. 14 to 16
C. 20 to 22
D. 26 to 28

28. In which one of the following holandric inheritances is seen?

A. Achondroplasia
B. Haemophilia
C. Hairy pinna
D. Phenylketonuria

29. All of the following are nucleolar chromosomes, EXCEPT:

A. 13
B. 15
C. 18
D. 21

30. Which chromosome represents the Barr body?

A. Active X
B. Active Y
C. Inactive X
D. Inactive Y

31. Which is the shortest chromosome?
  A. X
  B. Y
  C. 1
  D. 20

32. Which is the longest chromosome?
  A. 1
  B. 10
  C. X
  D. Y

33. On which chromosome locus for ABO gene is located?
  A. One
  B. Six
  C. Nine
  D. Sixteen

34. On which chromosome locus for Rh gene is located?
  A. One
  B. Six
  C. Nine
  D. Sixteen

35. On which chromosome locus for HLA gene is located?
  A. One
  B. Six
  C. Nine
  D. Sixteen

36. On which chromosome locus for blood group secretor gene is located?
  A. One
  B. Six
  C. Nine
  D. Nineteen

37. On which chromosome locus for heavy chain of immuno-globulin gene is located?
  A. Two
  B. Nine
  C. Fourteen
  D. Twenty two

38. On which chromosome locus kappa light chain of immuno-globulin gene is located?
  A. Two
  B. Nine
  C. Fourteen
  D. Twenty two

39. On which chromosome locus for lambda light chain of immunoglobulin gene is located?
  A. Two
  B. Nine
  C. Fourteen
  D. Twenty two

40. Which one of the following is the karyotype of Klinefelter's syndrome?
  A. 46 XY
  B. 47 XXY
  C. 45 X
  D. 47 XXX

41. Which chromosomal anomaly is present in Cri du chat syndrome?

A. del 5q
B. del 5p
C. del 7q
D. del 15q

42. All of the following are indications for prenatal diagnosis EXCEPT

A. Late maternal age
B. Sex determination
C. Risk of neural tube defect
D. Family history of some genetic defect

43. What type of inheritance is seen in AB blood group?

A. Dominant
B. Recessive
C. Codominant
D. Intermediate

44. What type of inheritance is seen in sickle cell trait?

A. Dominant
B. Recessive
C. Codominant
D. Intermediate

45. Robertsorian translocation involves two breaks near two centromeres of which of the following chromosomes?

A. Two metacentric
B. Two submetacentric
C. Two acrocentric
D. Metacentric and acrocentric

46. What type of inheritance is seen in thalassemia?

A. Autosomal dominant
B. Autosomal recessive
C. X linked recessive
D. X linked dominant

47. All of the following acrocentric chromosomes are with satellite, EXCEPT:

A. 13
B. 14
C. 22
D. Y

48. All of the following are acrocentric chromosomes, EXCEPT:

A. 15
B. 16
C. 21
D. Y

49. Approximately how many genes are present in human genome?

A. 46
B. 300
C. 3000
D. 30,000

50. Approximately how many protein coding genes are present in human genome?

A. 3000
B. 10,000
C. 27,000
D. 30,000

51. **Approximately how many RNA coding genes are present in human genome?**
    A. 3000
    B. 10,000
    C. 27,000
    D. 30,000

52. **Crossing over of chromosomes occurs during which one of the following?**
    A. Mitosis
    B. Meiosis
    C. Fertilization
    D. Transcription

53. **Karyotype analysis can be conducted on cells that have entered which one of the following stages of cell division?**
    A. Metaphase of meiosis I
    B. Metaphase of meiosis II
    C. Metaphase of mitosis
    D. Anaphase of mitosis

54. **Crossing over of chromosomes occurs during which stage of prophase of meiosis I?**
    A. Leptotene
    B. Zygotene
    B. Pachytene
    D. Diakinesis

55. **Which of the following is the origin of the mitochondrial DNA of all human adult cells?**
    A. Paternal only
    B. Maternal only
    C. Paternal and maternal
    D. Either paternal or maternal

56. **Which one of the following is often the preferred stage for more detailed cytogenetic analysis?**
    A. Meiotic prometaphase
    B. Meiotic metaphase
    C. Mitotic prometaphase
    D. Mitotic metaphase

57. **Most genetic metabolic diseases are caused by mutation in which one of the following?**
    A. Mitochondrial genes
    B. DNA repair genes
    C. Genes coding structural proteins
    D. Genes coding enzymes

58. **A child of a woman who is carrying D-G translocation, can have which one of the syndromes?**
    A. Down
    B. Turner
    C. Klinefelter
    D. Cri du chat

59. **All of the following contain 23 chromosomes, EXCEPT:**
    A. Primary oocyte
    B. Secondary oocyte
    C. First polar body
    D. Second polar body

60. In which one of the following Barr body is present?
A. Zygote
B. Morula
C. 10 days embryo
D. 16 days embryo

61. Which one of the following configurations of the karyotype indicates Robertsonian translocation?
A. A/D
B. B/D
C. C/D
D. D/G

62. What is the probability of having normal sons, if a man affected with X linked recessive disorder marries a normal woman?
A. 0%
B. 25%
C. 50%
D. 100%

63. Which one of the following, would be a possibility of progeny, if a woman with autosomal recessive disorder marries a normal man?
A. 25% carrier
B. All carrier
C. 50% normal 50% carrier
D. All affected

64. Which one of the following, would be a possibility of progeny, if an affected man with an autosomal recessive disorder marries a heterozygous carrier woman?
A. 25% children carrier
B. All carrier
C. 50% normal 50% affected
D. 50% affected, 50% carrier

65. Which one of the following, would be a possibility of progeny, if both parents are heterozygous for an autosomal dominant condition?
A. 25% normal, 75% affected
B. 75% normal, 25% affected
C. 50% normal, 50% affected
D. 50% affected, 50% carrier

66. Which one of the following, would be a possibility of progeny, if one parent is heterozygous for an autosomal dominant condition and the other is normal?
A. 25% normal, 75% affected
B. 75% normal, 25% affected
C. 50% normal, 50% affected
D. 50% affected, 50% carrier

67. Which one of the following, would be a possibility of progeny, if a man with X linked condition marries a normal woman?
A. All sons affected, all daughters carrier
B. All daughters carrier, all sons normal

   C. All daughters affected, all sons normal
   D. Both sons and daughters affected

68. **Which one of the following, would be a possibility of progeny, if a man with hemophilia marries a normal woman?**
   A. All sons affected, all daughters carrier
   B. All daughters carrier, all sons normal
   C. All daughters affected, sons normal
   D. Both sons and daughters affected

69. **Which one of the following traits is expressed only in homozygous state?**
   A. Autosomal dominant   B. Autosomal recessive
   C. X linked dominant   D. X linked recessive

70. **Which one of the following conditions is associated with raised levels of alfa fetoproteins in maternal serum?**
   A. Down's syndrome   B. Marfan's syndrome
   C. Hemophilia   D. Anencephaly

71. **Which one of the following conditions is associated with reduced levels of alfa fetoproteins in maternal serum?**
   A. Down's syndrome   B. Marfan's syndrome
   C. Hemophilia   D. Anencephaly

72. **All of the following are biochemical markers used in triple test of maternal serum for prenatal diagnosis of Down syndrome, EXCEPT:**
   A. Level of AFP reduced
   B. Level of AFP increased
   C. Level of HCG increased
   D. Level of unconjugate oestriol reduced

73. **During intrauterine life, when the Barr body appears in the extraembryonic membranes?**
   A. 12th day   B. 16th day
   C. 1st month   D. 2nd month

74. **During intrauterine life, when the Barr body appears in the cells of the embryo?**
   A. 12th day   B. 16th day
   C. 1st month   D. 2nd month

75. **Which one of the following inheritances follows the Mendel's laws?**
   A. Single gene   B. Mitochondrial
   C. Polygenic   D. Multifactorial

76. Which one of the following chromosomes is a gene rich chromosome?
   A. 4
   B. 18
   C. 22
   D. Y

77. Which one of the following chromosomes is a gene poor chromosome?
   A. 4
   B. 10
   C. 19
   D. 22

78. Which one of the following nitrogen containing base is present only in RNA?
   A. Adenine
   B. Guanine
   C. Cytosine
   D. Uracil

79. On which one of the following anticodons are located?
   A. rRNA
   B. tRNA
   C. mRNA
   D. miRNA

80. During which phase of cell cycle DNA is duplicated?
   A. G0
   B. G1
   C. G2
   D. S

81. Which one of the following the mechanism is responsible for genomic imprinting?
   A. Acetylation
   B. Phosphorylation
   C. Methylation
   D. Transposition

82. Which one of the following enzymes is utilized by stem cells and neoplastic cells to lengthen the telomeres?
   A. Topoisomerase
   B. Telomerase
   C. DNA ligase
   D. DNA polymerase

83. Which one of the following enzymes is not utilized by majority of normal cells so that chromosomes normally get successively shorter after each replication?
   A. Topoisomerase
   B. Telomerase
   C. DNA ligase
   D. DNA polymerase

84. Most genetic metabolic diseases are caused by mutations in which one of the following?
   A. DNA repair genes
   B. Mitochondrial genes
   C. Genes coding for structural proteins
   D. Genes coding for enzymes

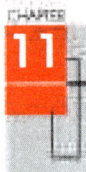

Radiology

1. **All of the following effects of X-rays form basis of radiography, EXCEPT:**
   A. Photographic
   B. Fluroscent
   C. Biological
   D. Resonance

2. **All of the following are properties of the X-rays EXCEPT:**
   A. Penetrating power
   B. Photographic effect
   C. Fluroscent effect
   D. Resonance

3. **X-rays are composed of particles of energy called:**
   A. Atoms
   B. Electrons
   C. Neutrons
   D. Photons

4. **What kind of waves are X-rays?**
   A. Sound
   B. Magnetic
   C. Electric
   D. Electromagnetic

5. **Which one of the following produces most radiopaque shadow on X-ray film?**
   A. Bone
   B. Cartilage
   C. Enamel
   D. Muscle

6. **Which one of the following is properties of the X-rays is used for therapeutic purpose?**
   A. Photographic
   B. Fluroscent
   C. Biological
   D. Penetrating power

7. **In a plain radiograph of thorax PA (posterior-anterior) view shadow of the right border of the heart is formed by all of the following, EXCEPT:**
   A. Superior vena cava
   B. Inferior vena cava
   C. Right atrium
   D. Right ventricle

8. **Hilar shadows seen in a plain radiograph of thorax PA (posterior-anterior) view comprise all of the following structures, EXCEPT:**
   A. Blood vessels
   B. Pleura
   C. Lymph nodes
   D. Bronchi

9. In a plain radiograph of thorax PA (posterior-anterior) view shadow of the left border of the heart is formed by all of the following, EXCEPT:

A. Aortic knuckle
B. Pulmonary conus
C. Left ventricle
D. Left atrium

10. All of the following are the common types of heart shadows seen in the plain radiograph PA view of the chest, EXCEPT:

A. Vertcal
B. Transverse
C. J shaped
D. Oblique

11. Which salt of barium is used for barium meal studies?

A. Carbonate
B. Chloride
C. Sulfate
D. Iodide

12. Barium sulfate is used as a contrast medium in radiological studies of gastrointestinal tract, because of its all of the following characteristics, EXCEPT:

A. Stable
B. Nontoxic
C. Soluble in water
D. Insoluble in water

13. A barium swallow shows the patients mid oesophagus compressed by a structure anterior to it. Which one of the following is responsible for it?

A. Right bronchus
B. Left ventricle
C. Right ventricle
D. Left atrium

14. How many milliliters of barium sulfate are used while doing Barium meal study?

A. 100
B. 200
C. 500
D. 1000

15. How many milliliters of barium sulfate are used while doing Barium enema study?

A. 200
B. 400
C. 600
D. 1000

16. During which days of menstrual cycle procedure of hysterosalpingography is done?

A. 1 to 5
B. 6 to 11
C. 14 to 20
D. 21 to 25

17. The radiological procedure for assessing the functional status of the kidney is called:

A. KUB film
B. Intravenous pyelography
C. Ascending pyelography
D. Micturating urethrogram

18. How many milliliters of contrast medium are used while doing hysterosalpingography?
    - A. 6–10
    - B. 10–12
    - C. 12–15
    - D. 15–16

19. Which one of the following is used in computerized axial tomography (CAT) scanning?
    - A. Sound waves
    - B. X rays
    - C. Radio waves
    - D. Radio-isotopes

20. How many degrees of rotation is allowed by a X-ray tube on the yoke, while doing computerized axial tomography (CAT) scanning?
    - A. 90
    - B. 180
    - C. 270
    - D. 360

21. Which one of the following is used in magnetic resonance imaging (MRI)?
    - A. Sound waves
    - B. X rays
    - C. Radio waves
    - D. Radio-isotopes

22. In magnetic resonance imaging (MRI), which one of the following is used in combination with magnetic field?
    - A. Sound waves
    - B. X rays
    - C. Radio waves
    - D. Radio-isotopes

23. All of the following are properties of the sound waves used in ultrasonography, EXCEPT:
    - A. High frequency
    - B. Transmitted in beams
    - C. Inaudible to humans
    - D. Pulses repeated about 100 times per second

24. Which one of the following is used in positron emission tomography (PET)
    - A. Sound waves
    - B. X-rays
    - C. Radio waves
    - D. Radio-isotopes

Medical Ethics

1. All of the following are principles of medical ethics, EXCEPT
   A. Justice
   B. Beneficence
   C. Autonomy
   D. Maleficience

2. While imparting informed choice, the patient is entitled for all of the following, EXCEPT:
   A. Information about all options
   B. Option of non-participation
   C. No vested interest
   D. Duress

3. What is the important element of a valid informed consent
   A. Disclosure of information
   B. Capacity of the subject to understand
   C. Voluntariness
   D. All of the above

4. All of the following are the criteria for population screening of carrier detection, EXCEPT:
   A. Infromed consent
   B. Confidentiality
   C. Full counseling
   D. Compulsory

5. In which one of the following stems cells for therapeutic cloning is not permissible?
   A. Animal human hybrid
   B. Embryo up to 14 days
   C. Umbilical cord
   D. Embryo of 30 days

6. In which of the following somatic cell gene therapy is not ethical issue?
   A. Treating serious disease
   B. To increase height
   C. To increase athletic prowess
   D. To alter intelligence

7. **When parents wish to do predictive genetic testing of their 7 years old son for an adult onset. Autosomal dominant disorder that runs in the family, which principle of medical ethics is at the risk of being compromised?**
   A. Justice
   B. Beneficence
   C. Autonomy
   D. Non-maleficence

8. **In which of the following termination of pregnancy would be a debatable issue?**
   A. Down syndrome
   B. Minor cleft palate
   C. Open neural tube defect
   D. Autism

9. **Which of the following may be unintended consequences of genetic population screening?**
   A. Stigmatization
   B. Adverse psychological consequences
   C. Discrimination at work place
   D. All of the above

10. **Prenatal sex determination is against which of the following principles of medical ethics?**
    A. Justice
    B. Beneficence
    C. Non-maleficence
    D. All of the above

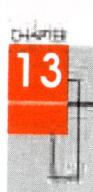
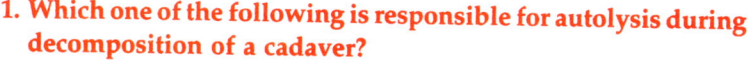

Embalming

1. Which one of the following is responsible for autolysis during decomposition of a cadaver?

A. Bacteria

B. Viruses

C. Magots

D. Own digestive enzymes

2. Which one of the following is responsible for bloating during decomposition of a cadaver?

A. Pus

B. Gas

C. Blood

D. Lymph

3. All of the following are natural means of preservation of a cadaver, EXCEPT:

A. Snow capped mountains

B. Extreme dry areas

C. Watery peat bogs

D. Evisceration

4. All of the following are artificial means of preservation of a cadaver, EXCEPT:

A. Refrigeration

B. Arterial injection

C. Watery peat bogs

D. Cavity injection

5. What is essential component of embalming solution?

A. Preservation

B. Restoration

C. Disinfection

D. All of the above

6. What is the basic goal of embalming?

A. Preservation

B. Presentation

C. Sanitization

D. All of the above

7. What is the role of crystals of thymol in embalming solution?

A. Fungicide

B. Bactericide

C. Stabilizer

D. Wetting agent

8. What is the role of glycerin in embalming solution?

A. Fungicide

B. Bactericide

C. Stabilizer

D. Wetting agent

9. What is the role of borax in embalming solution?
    A. Fungicide
    B. Bactericide
    C. Buffering agent
    D. Wetting agent

10. What is the role of methyl alcohol in embalming solution?
    A. Anticoagulant
    B. Buffering agent
    C. Stabilizer
    D. Wetting agent

11. What is the role of sodium citrate in embalming solution?
    A. Anticoagulant
    B. Buffering agent
    C. Stabilizer
    D. Wetting agent

12. In an embalming solution formalin plays an important role as all of the following, EXCEPT:
    A. Antiseptic
    B. Fixative
    C. Disinfectant
    D. Fungicide

Communication Skills and Attitude

1. What is the major component of medical learning, according Bloom's taxonomy?
   A. Knowledge
   B. Skills
   C. Attitude
   D. All of the above

2. What is the main component of attitude?
   A. Affective
   B. Cognitive
   C. Behavioral
   D. All of the above

3. All of the following are guidelines for effective communication, EXCEPT:
   A. Good listener
   B. Talk and talk
   C. Know your audience
   D. Avoid extremes

4. Which factors influence communication?
   A. Social
   B. Psychological
   C. Environmental
   D. All of the above

5. All of the following are basic foundations of good communication, EXCEPT:
   A. Credibility
   B. Content
   C. Context
   D. Complexity

6. All of the following factors can influence interpersonal relationship of doctor and patient, EXCEPT:
   A. Trust
   B. Empathy
   C. Superiority
   D. Autonomy

7. All of the following are the methods to overcome barriers of communication, EXCEPT:
   A. Be good listener
   B. Clarity in act
   C. Know your patient
   D. Using words having vague meaning

8. **All of the following are barriers of communications, EXCEPT:**
   - A. Cross cultural
   - B. Blood brain
   - C. Interpersonal
   - D. Perception

9. **All of the following 'Cs' form basic foundation of good communication, EXCEPT:**
   - A. Credibility
   - B. Content
   - C. Contrast
   - D. Context

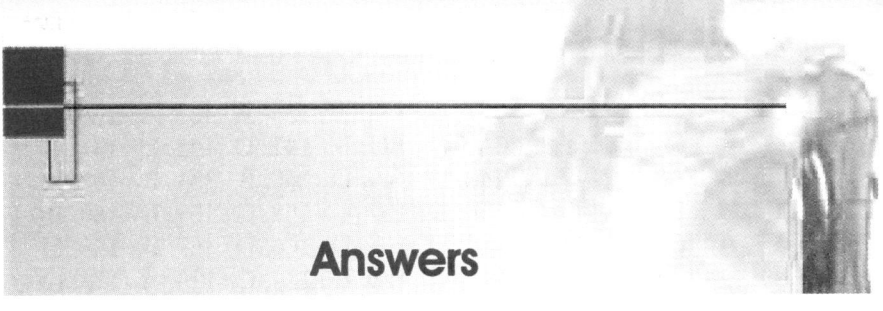

Answers

1. General Anatomy

1. D	2. C	3. C	4. C	5. B	6. B	7. B	8. C
9. A	10. B	11. C	12. A	13. D	14. A	15. D	16. A
17. D	18. A	19. B	20. C	21. B	22. A	23. C	24. A
25. A	26. B	27. A	28. C	29. B	30. B	31. A	32. A
33. A	34. D	35. B	36. C	37. A	38. B	39. C	40. C
41. C	42. B	43 B	44. B	45. C	46. C	47. A	48. D
49. B	50. C	51. D	52. D	53. D	54. C	55. B	56. D
57. A	58. D	59. D	60. B	61. D	62. D	63. A	64. B
65. B	66. D	67. C	68. D	69. D	70. A	71. D	72. D
73. B	74. B	75. C	76. B	77. D	78. C	79. C	80. A
81. D	82. C	83. C	84. D	85. D	86. A	87. B	88. B
89. A	90. A	91. C	92. C	93. A	94. D	95. B	96. A
97. C	98. B	99. D	100. A	101. D	102. A	103. B	104. D
105. B	106. D	107. D	108. C	109. D	110. B	111. D	112. B

2. Superior Extremity

1. B	2. A	3. C	4. C	5. B	6. C	7. B	8. A
9. D	10. B	11. C	12. A	13. D	14. D	15. D	16. C
17. D	18. D	19. A	20. D	21. C	22. C	23. A	24. C
25. A	26. C	27. A	28. B	29. D	30. B	31. C	32. C
33. D	34. A	35. C	36. B	37. B	38. A	39. A	40. B
41. A	42. B	43 D	44. B	45. D	46. B	47. A	48. D
49. B	50. C	51. B	52. A	53. A	54. D	55. A	56. B
57. B	58. C	59. D	60. B	61. B	62. B	63. C	64. D
65. D	66. B	67. B	68. A	69. C	70. B	71. C	72. C
73. A	74. D	75. B	76. D	77. A	78. A	79. B	80. B
81. D	82. D	83. D	84. C	85. A	86. D	87. B	88. C
89. D	90. A	91. A	92. B	93. D	94. B	95. C	96. B
97. B	98. A	99. A	100. C	101. C	102. D	103. C	104. A
105. D	106. D	107. C	108. A	109. B	110. D	111. D	112. C
113. D	114. D	115. B	116. A	117. B	118. B	119. B	120. B
121. A	122. B	123. A	124. B	125. B	126. D	127. A	128. B

129. A	130. A	131. A	132. B	134. D	134. A	135. A	136. C
137. B	138. B	139. B	140. D	141. B	142. D	143. D	144. C
145. C	146. C	147. A	148. D	149. D	150. B	151. B	152. A
153. D	154. A	155. C	156. C	157. C	158. C	159. D	160. B
161. A	162. C	163. D	164. D	165. D	166. D	167. B	168. D
169. B	170. A	171. A	172. C	173. B	174. C	175. A	176. D
177. B	178. D	179. B	180. C	181. D	182. B	183. D	184. D
185. A	186. B	187. B	188. B				

3. Inferior Extremity

1. B	2. C	3. C	4. C	5. B	6. C	7. B	8. B
9. C	10. A	11. D	12. B	13. D	14. B	15. B	16. A
17. C	18. C	19. B	20. A	21. C	22. C	23. D	24. A
25. C	26. C	27. D	28. A	29. D	30. B	31. A	32. C
33. B	34. B	35. C	36. B	37. C	38. C	39. B	40. D
41. D	42. D	43 A	44. D	45. C	46. A	47. B	48. D
49. C	50. B	51. C	52. C	53. C	54. D	55. B	56. D
57. C	58. B	59. B	60. A	61. C	62. B	63. B	64. A
65. B	66. B	67. C	68. A	69. C	70. D	71. C	72. C
73. D	74. A	75. A	76. B	77. B	78. B	79. B	80. B
81. A	82. A	83. C	84. B	85. A	86. D	87. D	88. C
89. D	90. B	91. C	92. D	93. D	94. D	95. B	96. D
97. B	98. D	99. D	100. D	101. D	102. B	103. B	104. C
105. B	106. D	107. A	108. D	109. B	110. C	111. A	112. A
113. B	114. A	115. A	116. B	117. B	118. A	119. D	120. D
121. A	122. B	123. D	124. C	125. B	126. B	127. A	128. A
129. D	130. C	131. B	132. C	133. D	134. D	135. B	136. C
137. D	138. D	139. C	140. D	141. A	142. A	143. B	144. B
145. C	146. A	147. C	148. B	149. C	150. D	151. D	152. D
153. D	154. A	155. D	156. B	157. D	168. B	159. C	160. D
161. C	162. D	163. D	164. C	165. B	166. D	167. C	168. C
169. C	170. A	171. B	172. D	173. D	174. B	175. C	

4. Thorax

1. B	2. D	3. B	4. B	5. C	6. A	7. A	8. D
9. A	10. A	11. B	12. D	13. B	14. C	15. C	16. C
17. B	18. B	19. B	20. C	21. B	22. C	23. B	24. B
25. A	26. B	27. D	28. B	29. A	30. D	31. B	32. C
33. C	34. B	35. D	36. C	37. D	38. A	39. B	40. C
41. B	42. B	43. B	44. C	45. C	46. D	47. D	48. C
49. A	50. D	51. C	52. B	53. C	54. D	55. D	56. B

57. A	58. B	59. D	60. B	61. D	62. D	63. D	64. A
65. D	66. B	67. C	68. B	69. B	70. B	71. D	72. B
73. C	74. D	75. B	76. C	77. A	78. D	79. C	80. C
81. D	82. C	83. B	84. B	85. C	86. A	87. C	88. B
89. D	90. D	91. D	92. B	93. D	94. D	95. B	96. D
97. C	98. D	99. A	100. B	101. D	102. B	103. B	104. A
105. B	106. C	107. D	108. A	109. B	110. C	111. A	112. C
113. D	114. B	115. C	116. D	117. C	118. B	119. B	120. B
121. D	122. A	123. B	124. C	125. C	126. B	127. A	128. D
129. B	130. A	131. D	132. A	134. B	134. D	135. C	136. A
137. B	138. D						

5. Abdomen

1. A	2. C	3. D	4. D	5. D	6. A	7. C	8. B
9. C	10. C	11. D	12. B	13. B	14. B	15. C	16. D
17. B	18. D	19. C	20. B	21. D	22. A	23. D	24. C
25. B	26. C	27. D	28. A	29. C	30. A	31. D	32. D
33. A	34. A	35. D	36. C	37. B	38. D	39. A	40. A
41. A	42. D	43. C	44. A	45. A	46. D	47. A	48. C
49. A	50. C	51. A	52. B	53. B	54. C	55. A	56. D
57. A	58. C	59. A	60. A	61. A	62. D	63. D	64. D
65. B	66. A	67. B	68. B	69. B	70. C	71. B	72. A
73. A	74. D	75. B	76. D	77. C	78. A	79. A	80. D
81. D	82. A	83. B	84. D	85. C	86. B	87. D	88. D
89. C	90. D	91. C	92. D	93. A	94. B	95. C	96. A
97. B	98. B	99. D	100. D	101. C	102. D	103. B	104. B
105. C	106. B	107. B	108. D	109. C	110. D	111. A	112. B
113. C	114. B	115. D	116. C	117. D	118. B	119. A	120. D
121. A	122. B	123. C	124. A	125. D	126. A	127. C	128. D
129. A	130. C	131. C	132. D	133. C	134. B	135. A	136. B
137. C	138. D	139. A	140. D	141. D	142. B	143. C	144. C
145. D	146. C	147. B	148. C	149. D	150. D	151. D	152. D
153. A	154. D	155. C	156. D	157. D	158. A	159. B	160. C
161. C	162. C	163. C	164. D	165. A	166. D	167. D	168. B
169. D	170. C	171. C	172. A	173. B	174. B	175. B	176. D
177. D	178. D	179. B	180. D	181. B	182. A	183. D	184. B
185. D	186. B	187. D	188. D	189. C	190. B	191. C	192. A
193. B	194. A	195. D	196. A	197. B	198. B	199. B	200. D
201. C	202. B	203. C	204. A	205. B	206. B	207. D	208. D

6. Head, Face and Neck

1. C	2. A	3. C	4. B	5. A	6. B	7. B	8. A
9. A	10. D	11. D	12. A	13. A	14. B	15. B	16. D
17. C	18. C	19. B	20. D	21. C	22. D	23. A	24. C
25. A	26. D	27. A	28. B	29. A	30. B	31. A	32. C
33. D	34. C	35. D	36. B	37. B	38. D	39. D	40. D
41. B	42. D	43. C	44. C	45. A	46. B	47. D	48. B
49. C	50. D	51. D	52. B	53. C	54. B	55. C	56. C
57. D	58. C	59. A	60. C	61. B	62. B	63. B	64. C
65. B	66. D	67. C	68. A	69. A	70. B	71. C	72. A
73. B	74. C	75. B	76. A	77. B	78. C	79. B	80. D
81. B	82. B	83. C	84. A	85. A	86. C	87. B	88. D
89. B	90. D	91. C	92. C	93. A	94. A	95. B	96. B
97. C	98. B	99. D	100. A	101. C	102. A	103. D	104. D
105. D	106. C	107. C	108. C	109. A	110. C	111. D	112. B
113. D	114. C	115. D	116. A	117. B	118. B	119. C	120. A
121. D	122. B	123. C	124. B	125. B	126. D	127. C	128. D
129. D	130. A	131. A	132. B	133. C	134. C	135. C	136. B
137. C	138. C	139. B	140. B	141. B	142. D	143. C	144. B
145. B	146. C	147. B	148. D	149. C	150. B	151. C	152. A
153. C	154. C	155. D	156. A	157. D	158. A	159. C	160. B
161. C	162. A	163. D	164. D	165. C	166. D	167. B	168. D
169. A	170. B	171. C	172. D	173. D	174. B	175. B	176. C
177. D	178. C	179. B	180. C	181. A	182. C	183. B	184. A
185. D	186. B	187. D	188. B	189. B	190. D	191. C	192. B
193. C	194. D	195. A	196. D	197. D	198. A	199. B	200. B
201. D	202. A	203. D	204. B	205. A	206. D	207. C	208. D
209. B	210. B	211. A	212. C	213. D	214. C	215. C	216. C
217. C	218. A	219. C	220. D	221. D	222. A	223. A	224. C
225. B	226. D	227. C	228. A	229. B	230. D	231. B	232. B
233. C	234. B	235. C	236. D	237. B	238. B	239. C	240. D
241. B	242. C	243. B	244. C	245. B	246. C	247. C	248. B
249. B	250. C	251. D	252. D	253. D	254. B	255. D	256. D
257. C	258. B	259. D					

7. Brain

1. A	2. B	3. D	4. A	5. A	6. D	7. B	8. C
9. B	10. B	11. C	12. D	13. C	14. C	15. D	16. B
17. D	18. C	19. D	20. B	21. D	22. C	23. A	24. B
25. B	26. C	27. B	28. C	29. C	30. C	31. D	32. B
33. D	34. C	35. A	36. B	37. B	38. C	39. C	40. D

41. C	42. D	43. A	44. C	45. A	46. D	47. B	48. B
49. C	50. C	51. B	52. B	53. C	54. A	55. C	56. C
57. B	58. A	59. B	60. B	61. C	62. A	63. D	64. D
65. D	66. A	67. C	68. D	69. C	70. B	71. B	72. A
73. B	74. A	75. C	76. B	77. A	78. D	79. C	80. C
81. A	82. A	83. B	84. A	85. B	86. B	87. A	88. D
89. A	90. B	91. C	92. D	93. B	94. D	95. D	96. A
97. B	98. C	99. D	100. D	101. D	102. C	103. B	104. B
105. B	106. A	107. D	108. D	109. D	110. D	111. A	112. C
113. A	114. C	115. D	116. A	117. C	118. B	119. A	120. B
121. B	122. D	123. C	124. B	125. B	126. C	127. A	128. B
129. D	130. A	131. A	132. D	134. A	134. B	135. D	136. D
137. B	138. D	139. C	140. A	141. A	142. B	143. A	144. D
145. C	146. C	147. A	148. D	149. A	150. D	151. B	152. D
153. B	154. B	155. A	156. A	157. B	158. C	159. D	160. A
161. D	162. B	163. B	164. B	165. A	166. A	167. A	168. A
169. A	170. B	171. D	172. D	173. D	174. A	175. C	176. B
177. A	178. C	179. D	180. D	181. C	182. D	183. B	184. D
185. D	186. B	187. D	188. D	189. B	190. C	191. D	192. C
193. D	194. A	195. D	196. D	197. A	198. B	199. A	200. C

8. Embryology

1. C	2. D	3. B	4. A	5. A	6. B	7. B	8. C
9. B	10. D	11. D	12. C	13. B	14. C	15. A	16. C
17. A	18. C	19. B	20. B	21. B	22. B	23. C	24. C
25. C	26. C	27. A	28. C	29. B	30. C	31. C	32. B
33. D	34. C	35. D	36. C	37. B	38. A	39. B	40. B
41. A	42. C	43. A	44. C	45. B	46. C	47. A	48. B
49. D	50. A	51. B	52. B	53. A	54. A	55. A	56. C
57. B	58. C	59. A	60. D	61. B	62. C	63. C	64. A
65. A	66. A	67. B	68. C	69. B	70. B	71. A	72. B
73. D	74. D	75. B	76. B	77. A	78. A	79. B	80. B
81. D	82. A	83. B	84. D	85. B	86. D	87. D	88. B
89. B	90. D	91. A	92. A	93. D	94. A	95. B	96. B
97. B	98. C	99. D	100. B	101. D	102. B	103. B	104. A
105. D	106. D	107. B	108. B	109. C	110. D	111. C	112. A
113. D	114. B	115. A	116. D	117. D	118. C	119. A	120. B
121. B	122. A	123. D	124. D	125. C	126. B	127. C	128. D
129. C	130. C	131. B	132. C	134. D	134. D	135. C	136. D
137. C	138. D	139. A	140. A	141. B	142. D	143. D	144. D
145. A	146. C	147. D	148. A	149. C	150. A	151. B	152. A

153. A 154. C 155. C 156. C 157. A 158. B 159. C 160. B
161. A 162. D 163. A 164. D 165. B 166. C 167. B 168. D
169. A 170. B 171. D 172. C 173. B 174. D 175. C 176. A
177. C 178. C 179. D 180. D 181. B 182. D 183. D 184. B
185. C 186. A 187. C 188. B 189. A 190. B 191. C 192. B
193. B 194. D 195. B 196. C 197. A 198. D 199. B 200. A
201. B 202. B 203. B 204. A 205. B 206. B 207. D 208. D
209. D 210. C 211. D 212. B 213. D 214. B 215. A 216. D
217. A 218. D 219. B 220. C 221. D 222. A 223. C 224. B
225. C 226. C 227. D 228. D 229. B 230. B 231. A 232. A
233. C 234. C 235. A 236. B 237. D 238. B 239. D 240. D
241. B 242. B 243. D 244. B 245. C 246. C 247. A 248. C
249. D 250. C 251. A 252. B 253. D 254. A 255. B 256. C
257. D 258. B 259. C 260. B 261. B 262. A 263. D 264. D
265. D 266. C

9. Histology

  1. C   2. D   3. B   4. A   5. C   6. A   7. A   8. D
  9. C   10. D   11. A   12. A   13. D   14. B   15. A   16. A
 17. C   18. C   19. B   20. A   21. B   22. A   23. B   24. B
 25. B   26. B   27. D   28. D   29. B   30. A   31. D   32. C
 33. A   34. A   35. C   36. D   37. C   38. C   39. C   40. C
 41. B   42. C   43. A   44. A   45. A   46. A   47. D   48. B
 49. B   50. C   51. D   52. C   53. C   54. C   55. B   56. A
 57. D   58. B   59. B   60. B   61. A   62. D   63. B   64. C
 65. C   66. B   67. B   68. B   69. D   70. D   71. A   72. C
 73. A   74. C   75. B   76. D   77. C   78. A   79. B   80. D
 81. C   82. C   83. D   84. B   85. B   86. C   87. A   88. C
 89. D   90. A   91. A   92. D   93. B   94. C   95. D   96. C
 97. C   98. B   99. C 100. C 101. A 102. D 103. D 104. B
105. C 106. C 107. A 108. A 109. B 110. B 111. A 112. C
113. D 114. A 115. D 116. A 117. C 118. A 119. A 120. B
121. C 122. B 123. B 124. C 125. C 126. D 127. D 128. B
129. D 130. D 131. B 132. B 134. B 134. A 135. D 136. B
137. B 138. A 139. A 140. D 141. D 142. A 143. A 144. C
145. C 146. B 147. D 148. B 149. C 150. A 151. D 152. A
153. A 154. A 155. B 156. B 157. A 158. D 159. B 160. D
161. A 162. A 163. A 164. B 165. D 166. A 167. B 168. A
169. B 170. B 171. C 172. B 173. C 174. D 175. A 176. D
177. A 178. C 179. A 180. B 181. D 182. D 183. C 184. A
185. C 186. C 187. C 188. B 189. A 190. B

10. Genetics

1. A	2. B	3. C	4. B	5. B	6. A	7. C	8. C
9. A	10. B	11. C	12. D	13. C	14. A	15. D	16. C
17. B	18. C	19. B	20. B	21. A	22. C	23. B	24. B
25. A	26. B	27. B	28. C	29. C	30. C	31. B	32. A
33. C	34. A	35. B	36. D	37. C	38. A	39. D	40. B
41. B	42. B	43. C	44. D	45. C	46. B	47. D	48. B
49. D	50. C	51. A	52. B	53. C	54. B	55. B	56. C
57. D	58. A	59. A	60. D	61. D	62. A	63. C	64. D
65. A	66. C	67. C	68. B	69. B	70. D	71. A	72. B
73. A	74. B	75. A	76. C	77. A	78. D	79. B	80. D
81. C	82. B	83. B	84. D				

11. Radiology

1. D	2. D	3. D	4. D	5. C	6. C	7. D	8. B
9. D	10. C	11. C	12. C	13. B	14. B	15. D	16. B
17. B	18. A	19. B	20. D	21. C	22. C	23. D	24. D

12. Medial Ethics

1. D	2. D	3. D	4. D	5. D	6. A	7. C	8. B
9. D	10. D						

13. Embalming

1. D	2. B	3. D	4. C	5. D	6. D	7. A	8. D
9. C	10. C	11. A	12. D				

14. Communication Skills and Attitude

1. D	2. D	3. B	4. D	5. D	6. C	7. D	8. B
9. C							